CANCER BIOLOGY. II
Etiology and Therapy

CANCER BIOLOGY. II
Etiology and Therapy

Edited by

Cecilia M. Fenoglio, M.D.
Donald West King, M.D.

College of Physicians and Surgeons of Columbia University
New York

Based on a series of lectures presented at the
Given Institute of Pathobiology of the University of
Colorado in Aspen, Colorado, July 1975

Stratton Intercontinental Medical Book Corp. / New York

Courses Sponsored by the Given Institute, 1976

PUBLISHED IN THIS SERIES TO DATE

1. Fenoglio CM, Borek C, King DW (Eds): Cell Membranes—Structure, Receptors, and Transport (1975)
2. Pascal RR, Silva F, King DW (Eds): Cancer Biology, I—Induction, Regulation, Immunology and Therapy (1976)
3. Fenoglio CM, Goodman R, King DW (Eds): Developmental Genetics (1976)
4. Fenoglio CM, King DW (Eds): Cancer Biology, II—Etiology and Therapy (1976)
5. Borek C, King DW (Eds): Cancer Biology, III—Herpes Virus (1976)

ADVANCES IN PATHOBIOLOGY is published
under the general Series Editorship of
Dr. Donald West King.

Copyright © 1976
Stratton Intercontinental Medical Book Corp.
381 Park Avenue South
New York, N.Y. 10016

LC 75-3356. ISBN 0-913258-41-5
Printed in U.S.A.

CONTENTS

Contributors

Joseph H. Burchenal, M.D., Memorial Sloan-Kettering Cancer Center, New York, N.Y.

Judah Folkman, M.D., Department of Surgery, Harvard Medical School, Children's Hospital Medical Center, Boston, Mass.

Robert C. Gallo, M.D., Laboratory of Tumor Cell Biology, National Cancer Institute, Bethesda, Md.

Howard Green, M.D., Department of Biology, Massachusetts Institute of Technology, Cambridge, Mass.

Kevin Lafferty, M.D., National University of Canberra, Canberra, Australia

Elliot Osserman, M.D., Department of Medicine, Institute for Cancer Research, College of Physicians and Surgeons of Columbia University, New York, N.Y.

Janet D. Rowley, M.D., Department of Medicine, University of Chicago, Chicago, Ill.

Richard T. Smith, M.D., Department of Pathology, University of Florida College of Medicine, Gainesville, Fla.

George J. Todaro, M.D., Viral Leukemia and Lymphoma Branch, National Cancer Institute, Bethesda, Md.

Peter K. Vogt, Ph.D., Department of Microbiology, University of Southern California, Los Angeles, Calif.

I. Bernard Weinstein, M.D., Institute for Cancer Research, College of Physicians and Surgeons of Columbia University, New York, N.Y.

Foreword

The Cancer Biology seminar held in Aspen July 20–25, 1975 was supported by the National Cancer Institute under Grant #5R13 CA 15961-02. It is clear that multiple etiologic factors are important in the development of cancer, including viral, immunologic, hormonal and environmental (physical and chemical) agents. Cancer is a complex disease with multifactorial ramifications, and its etiology cannot be a simple one.

A strong emphasis on environmental factors has been emphasized in this conference; the study of viruses has contributed greatly to molecular and cellular biology and may play an important role in the etiology of leukemia. The participants, both those in basic biology research and those in clinical practice, emphasize the necessity for close cooperation as they approach the problems of etiology, diagnosis and treatment.

Donald West King

Introduction

The problems of etiology, diagnosis and therapy in cancer are enormous. Each field has its own specialized vocabulary, impeding communication between workers in different specialized areas. This monograph is the proceedings of an interdisciplinary seminar and as such may be of help to individuals holding single pieces of the enormous cancer puzzle.

Much of this seminar emphasizes external factors (viruses and carcinogens) which may play a role in the etiology of cancer. However, it is necessary to take a step away from the problem of neoplasia and define the growth controls which exist for non-neoplastic cells. Only then can we hope to determine if normal regulatory controls are present, absent or altered in neoplastic cell populations.

It is clear that external factors do have a regulatory function on the growth of the normal cell, and these factors affect various cells differently. (An example would be the lymphocyte mitogens which affect different classes of lymphocytes differently.) This differential response of cells to external stimuli would suggest that regulatory factors differ from one cell type to another; one would expect that disruption of these growth regulatory factors would result in a cancer of a single cell type.

These regulating systems are explored and defined by Howard Green, using the resting and growing state of the fibroblast as a model. He notes that as the cell shifts from the resting to growing state following mitogenic stimuli there is an increase in the protein synthetic machinery. This is reversible following withdrawal of the stimuli. The cellular regulation of the various components of the synthetic machinery differs, i.e., the regulation of the synthesis of mRNA and ribosomes differs. Replication of the genome also occurs following mitogenic stimuli; these features of cell growth are explored in the third volume of *Advances in Pathobiology.**

Clearly one group of external stimuli affecting cell growth is viruses. By applying some of the technics discussed in *Advances in Pathobiology 3, Developmental Genetics,* to the genetics of the RNA tumor viruses, fingerprints of mutant RNA, sequencing of RNA with localization of specific oligonucleotides of the genome and an analysis of DNA transcription may lead to advances in elucidating a possible viral etiology of cancer. The genome of these viruses can be studied using conditional and nonconditional viral mutants which represent deletions of the genetic material. This aspect

---

* A listing of the volumes in this series so far published is given on the verso of the title page of this book.

1

is discussed by Peter Vogt, who uses three functional classes of viral mutants. These mutants are defective in their ability to transform cells, to replicate in cells or to both transform and replicate in cells.

The RNA viruses are further explored in the discussions by Todaro and Gallo. Todaro points out that viral genetic material becomes incorporated into the host's own genetic machinery and then is transmitted with the host genes. These fragments of foreign genetic material (virogenes) which are normally repressed may become activated by intrinsic (genetic or hormonal) or extrinsic (chemical or viral) factors and lead to neoplastic growth.

Viral genes from one group of animals can lead to infective particles which can integrate into the DNA of other species and become part of the germ line, thus providing a mechanism by which stable interspecies transfer of genetic information can occur. The type C viruses are uniquely suited to this role, since they must incorporate into the host cellular DNA to replicate and they do not kill the cells they infect. The role of the type C RNA virus as a causative agent in leukemia is discussed by Gallo. He briefly surveys the problems encountered in trying to document proof that viruses are tumorogenic. He then details the replication and classification of these RNA viruses and concludes his discussion with the relationship of type C virus to human leukemia using a variety of experimental approaches.

A discussion of the viral etiology of cancer would be incomplete without a consideration of the DNA viruses. This subject is taken up at length in the following monograph, *Advances in Pathobiology 5.*

Another widely recognized group of external stimuli affecting cellular growth is a variety of chemical compounds. This aspect of etiology is presented in this monograph (also in no. 2 of the series) by Dr. Weinstein. In an historical survey he points out that in the 18th century, Sir Percival Potts demonstrated that coal tars were associated with human cancers and yet, in the 1970's, there are still 80,000 deaths a year from lung cancer—also related to coal tars. He surveys the current environmental situation, occupational and otherwise and points out that transplacental transport of certain compounds may affect the fetus. Following this background discussion he tackles the problem of how a chemical may serve as a carcinogen.

That viruses and chemicals do have effects on cells is well recognized, but undoubtedly these are only a fraction of a whole host of external factors which do. It is fascinating that something as simple as the geometric configuration of cells may also regulate their growth. This area is explored here by Folkman, who finds that growth in the two dimensional plane is virtually unlimited, whereas three dimensional growth is not. He relates this to a prime factor (vascularity) and ultimately to the cells' ability to obtain oxygen and nutrients and excrete wastes.

In considering etiologic agents of disease, it would be naive to discount genetic susceptibilities, but the relative importance of genetic versus environmental factors probably differs in each tumor. It is of interest that cells from tumors associated with specific etiologic agents have consistent chromosomal abnormalities (i.e., Burkitt's), whereas cells from tumors without specific etiologies have variable chromosomal alterations. These aspects of cancer biology are defined by Dr. Rowley.

Not only do external and genetic factors affect the mode of cellular growth but they may alter the cell membrane and produce characteristic antigenic changes (see *Advances in Pathobiology, no. 1*). These changes in cellular antigenicity provoke an immune response in the host, summarized here by Richard Smith, and, in an earlier volume, by John Marchalonis (*Advances in Pathobiology, no. 2*). In his overview, Dr. Smith deals with the nature of tumor antigens and the response they evoke in the host. These interactions are complex and involve an interaction between the tumor and the host defense systems. Different parts of this interaction may be duplicated in the laboratory but are less clear in the *in vivo* situation.

One of the initial problems in mounting an immunologic attack is the recognition of an intruder as a foreigner. As simple as one would think this would be, it is becoming evident that both a responding cell and a stimulating cell are required for such an identification to be made. The nature of the interaction and cooperation of these two types of cells (T lymphocytes and macrophages) are discussed by Dr. Lafferty.

In addition to the cellular effect on tumors, there is a host of soluble factors which may also have regulatory functions. Humoral antibody is certainly a major example of one of these (discussed by Dr. Smith), and lysozyme is now emerging as another important soluble mediator of cellular function. Dr. Osserman discusses the regulation of the effector function of macrophages by this material and compares it to the role of immunoglobulin on plasma cells.

By applying all that we know of etiologic factors and host responsiveness to tumors, we may hope in the future to better alter this response in a way which is beneficial to a given patient. However, preventive measures are not a reality for those already suffering from cancer. Fortunately for those people, significant advances have been made in cancer chemotherapy and these are summarized by Dr. Burchenal.

The continued close cooperation of cell biologists, virologists, endocrinologists, immunologists and clinicians will allow knowledge in one field to be available and applied in other fields. We may then be closer to the possibility of preventing and/or curing the disease most people fear.

The Editors

The Resting and Growing States of the Fibroblast

Howard Green, M.D.

What is greatly needed in the field of fundamental cancer research is some knowledge of how normal cells grow. Without it, the identification of causes of cancer (whether simple chemicals, viral genes or their products, or ionizing radiation) cannot be followed by any real progress with regard to their mechanism of action. This state of affairs has not prevented the development of successful therapy for some kinds of cancer, but it is difficult to imagine a general understanding of the disease and its therapy without detailed knowledge of the process of normal cell growth and its control.

The problem of cell growth can be conveniently divided into two parts. The first consists of the external regulating factors (mitogens or antimitogens) and their interaction with the target cells. In order that the growth of each differentiated cell type be regulated independently, these factors must be different for each cell type. Disruption of the basis for this part of the growth regulating mechanism should produce a cancer of only a single cell type. For example, specific chromosomal rearrangements such as those recently demonstrated in certain human leukemias lead to tumors of a single cell type. Presumably, the rearrangement affects a locus involved in the growth regulation of that cell type, but the same chromosomal rearrangement occurring in other cell types would produce no comparable disturbance.

A similar effect is probably responsible for the loss of neoplastic properties which occurs in the progeny of malignant teratoma cells. The process of differentiation evidently substitutes an intact regulating system characteristic of the differentiated cell type for the damaged one of the malignant stem cell. In this way, the process of differentiation leads to loss of neoplastic character.

The second part of the growth control system comes into operation after reception of the external growth controlling stimuli and prepares the cell for division or for the resting state. It seems likely that different cell types will

From the Department of Biology, Massachusetts Institute of Technology, Cambridge, Mass.

4

have much the same mechanism for this part of the control system. In most cells, division follows automatically at an interval following replication of the genome, so that preparation for division is really preparation for DNA synthesis. Except for a small minority of cell types, once DNA synthesis has begun, the cell cannot reach a new resting state until it has completed DNA synthesis and divided.

In no case known does a mitogenic stimulus act by directly initiating DNA synthesis. The same is true of oncogenic viruses. A mitogenic stimulus acts in such a way that the target cell changes its biosynthetic pattern from that characteristic of the resting state to that characteristic of the growing state. DNA synthesis usually begins only after 11–24 hours of stimulation, depending on the cell type. In order to understand the mitogenic response, it is necessary to ask what are the changes that prepare the cell for DNA synthesis. For the fibroblast stimulated by serum, to pass from resting to growing state, these changes are summarized in Table 1. The three major components of the protein-synthesizing machinery increase in amount during the transition [8,19]. The amounts of ribosomes and tRNA increase proportionally, so that the ratio between the two is the same in resting as in growing cells. For 3T6 cells the ratio is about 25 molecules of tRNA per ribosome. Other mammalian cell lines may have a lower ratio (for V79 cells it is 18:1 [Mauck and Green, unpublished]), but for a line in which resting and growing states can be compared, the ratio is unchanged. This is quite different from the behavior of these two components in bacteria (Table 2). While bacteria regulate their ribosome content according to their growth rate, they do not regulate their tRNA content in this way; as a result, tRNA content is in excess at low growth rates [12]. It may be postulated that it is advantageous for the mammalian cell, which must be able to

TABLE 1. Increase in Components of the Protein-Synthesizing Machinery in Growing as Compared with Resting Cells

Component	Amount of Increase per Unit of DNA	Origin of Increase
ribosomes	1.6–2.5 fold	increased formation decreased destruction
tRNA	same as for ribosomes	increased formation decreased destruction
mRNA	greater than for ribosomes and tRNA (2.3–4.0 fold)	increased formation no decrease in destruction

TABLE 2. Number of Transfer RNA Molecules per Ribosome

(a) *In Salmonella growing at different rates* (*data of O. Maaloe and N. O. Kjeldgaard* [12])

Doubling time	Transfer RNA molecules per ribosome
25 min.	15.5
50 min.	41
100 min.	64
300 min.	159

(b) *In mammalian fibroblast line 3T6*

resting	25
growing (Td = 15 hrs.)	25

maintain a resting state for long periods, to avoid the burden of an excess of tRNA.

Growing cells also contain more poly A(+) mRNA than resting cells [8]; as the difference is greater than for ribosomes, the ratio of mRNA to ribosomes in the growing state is higher by 50% or more. This change in ratio takes place quite early during the transition from resting to growing state, and is a convenient way of defining the boundary between the G_0 and G_1 states (Fig. 1).

The source of the increase in the various components is shown in Table 1. There is an increase in the rate of formation of all components during transition from resting to growing state. In addition, ribosomes and tRNA are more stable in growing than in resting cells (Table 3), so that conservation

TABLE 3. Lifetime of Cytoplasmic RNA of Resting 3T3 and 3T6 Cells

	Half-time	
	Resting	Growing
tRNA	36 hr	60 hr
rRNA 18S	70 hr	∞
28S	50 hr	∞
mRNA, poly(A)(+)	9 hr	9 hr

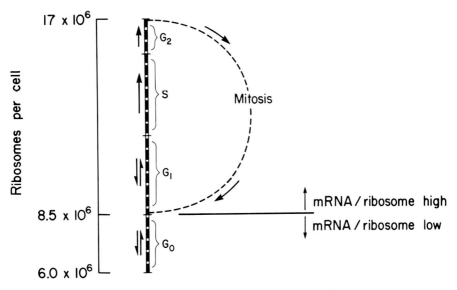

FIG. 1. The Division Cycle and the Resting State (G_0)

contributes to their accumulation in growing cells [1]. There is no difference between resting and growing cells in the stability of poly A($+$) mRNA (1), so the increased content of growing cells must be due entirely to a greater rate of formation.

The origins of the increased rate of formation of the three components are summarized in Table 4. The rates of transcription of pre-rRNA and pre-tRNA increase very quickly when resting fibroblasts are stimulated to prepare for division [4,13,14]. On the other hand, the over-all rate of transcription of HnRNA, the precursor of cytoplasmic mRNA, does not increase during transition from resting to growing state [13]; this rate is fixed in relation to the amount of DNA. In other cell types the amount of RNA polymerase II has been found to be much less subject to change than the amount of polymerase I [16]. The mitogen-stimulated lymphocyte appears to be exceptional for it increases appreciably its level of polymerase

TABLE 4. Over-all Transcription Rates (per unit of DNA) of Major Classes of RNA during Transition of 3T6 Cells from Resting State to the Initiation of DNA Synthesis

preribosomal RNA	increased
pretransfer RNA	increased
HnRNA	not increased

II, though not as much as that of polymerase I [7]. How the increase in enzyme activity is related to the rate of nucleoplasmic transcription in that cell type is not yet clear.

The increase in mRNA content required for growth is achieved in the fibroblast by an increase in the amount of HnRNA converted to mRNA. This conclusion is based on the following:

(1) Pulse-chase labeling of nuclear poly A shows that a greater fraction of this poly A emerges into the cytoplasm in growing cells [9].

(2) Kinetic analysis shows that while about 4% of poly A(+) HnRNA is converted to cytoplasmic mRNA in growing cells, the corresponding value for resting cells is less than half as large [11].

By a different kind of analysis, similar changes have been shown by Cooper to take place in the mitogen-stimulated lymphocyte [5].

The changes induced by a mitogenic stimulus and resulting in a buildup

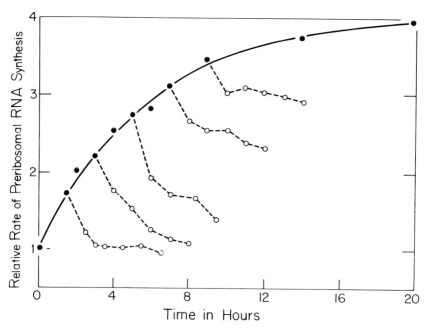

FIG. 2. Rate of Preribosomal RNA Synthesis after Withdrawal of Serum Stimulus. Solid line and solid circles show the increase in rate of synthesis after addition of serum-rich medium to resting 3T6 cultures at time zero. Open circles and hatched lines show the decline in rate when the serum-rich medium was removed and the original was replaced. Measurements of rate of incorporation of tritiated UTP were made after detergent treatment and in the presence of α amanitin at 0.25 μg/ml to suppress HnRNA synthesis (data of Mostafapour and Green [15]).

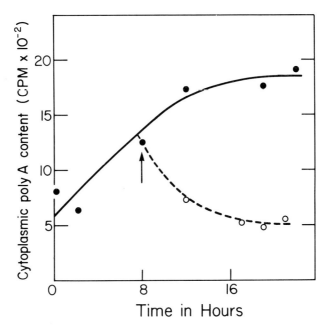

FIG. 3. Decline in Cytoplasmic Poly A Content after Withdrawal of Serum. Solid line and solid circles show rise in cytoplasmic poly A content after serum stimulation. Open circles and hatched line show decline in poly A content after withdrawal of the high serum medium (arrow). Measurements were made by hybridization of the poly A with tritiated poly U (data of Mostafapour and Green [15]).

of the protein-synthesizing machinery are reversed following withdrawal of the stimulus, but the rates of the reversal are different for the different components. Figure 2 shows the effect on pre-rRNA synthesis of withdrawing serum after varying periods of stimulation. In less than 30 minutes there was a definite drop in the synthetic rate. On the other hand, especially after long periods of serum stimulation, it required a long time for the rate to decline to the resting level. As in the case of the increase due to serum stimulation, a response begins quickly, but there is considerable inertia in the system and it may require many hours for the cell to reach a new equilibrium rate [15].

As would be expected from its behavior during shiftup following mitogenic stimulation, cytoplasmic poly A(+) mRNA content is adjusted downward more rapidly than ribosome content after withdrawal of the serum stimulus. Figure 3 shows the results of measurement of cytoplasmic poly A content (a good measure of poly A(+) mRNA content) following introduction and withdrawal of a serum stimulus. Within 8 hours after serum stimulation, 3T6 cells more than doubled their cytoplasmic poly A content. Within 8 hours of withdrawal of the serum stimulus the cytoplasmic poly A content declined to the resting level. The rate of this decline can be compared with that of the cytoplasmic ribosomes (measured as total RNA (Fig. 4)). The return of mRNA content to the resting level is considerably faster [15]. This is likely due to the fact that mRNA turns over much more rapidly than ribosomes (Table 3).

These experiments show that the cell regulates its mRNA content differently from that of its ribosomes. This has the advantage that the rate of protein synthesis can be adjusted more rapidly than ribosome content. In simple transitions between resting and growing state the rate of protein synthesis follows mRNA content much more closely than ribosome content [8,15], though under more severe shiftdown conditions it is possible for cells to reduce their rate of utilization of existing mRNA [2,3,6,17,18].

Changes in mRNA content can take place in the absence of ribosome synthesis. Resting 3T6 cells stimulated by serum in the presence of fluoro-

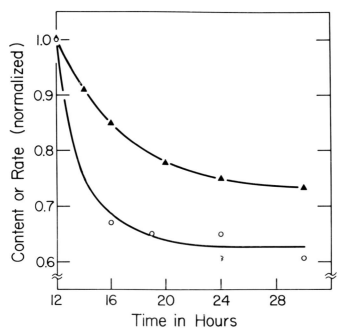

FIG. 4. Comparison of Declines of Ribosome and mRNA Content after Withdrawal of a Serum Stimulus. Circles, cytoplasmic poly A content; triangles, total cellular RNA (data of Mostafapour and Green [15]).

uridine are prevented by the drug from synthesizing ribosomes, but they nevertheless increase their cytoplasmic mRNA content [10].

Relations between the different parts of the program which prepares for growth can be studied by the use of mutants which cannot carry out a specific part of the program. For example, temperature-sensitive mutants in ribosomal RNA synthesis or aminoacylation of tRNA are known and could be employed for this purpose. Among the cell cycle mutants, those which result in failure of the cells to synthesize DNA are sometimes referred to as mutants for the initiation of DNA synthesis. This designation is likely to be incorrect in most cases. Any mutation which interferes with preparations for DNA synthesis will arrest the cell in the G_0 period, but from the complexity of these preparations it is obvious that most of these mutations will be unrelated to the DNA replication process. Study of such mutants may bring to light interesting aspects of the preparative program.

REFERENCES

1. Abelson HT, Johnson LF, Penman S, Green H: Cell 1: 161, 1974.
2. Baenziger NL, Jacobi CH, Tach RE: J Biol Chem 299: 3483, 1974.
3. Bandman E, Gurney T Jr: Exp Cell Res 90: 159, 1975.
4. Bombik BM, Baserga R: Proc Natl Acad Sci USA 71 2038, 1974.
5. Cooper HL: *In* Clarkson B and Baserga R (Eds): Control of Proliferation in Animal Cells, Cold Spring Harbor Conferences on Cell Proliferation, Vol. 1: 1974, p 769–783.
6. Engelhardt DL: J Cell Physiol 78: 333, 1971.
7. Jaehning JA, Stewart CC, Roeder RG: Cell 4: 51, 1975.
8. Johnson LF, Abelson HT, Green H, Penman S: Cell 1: 95, 1974.
9. Johnson LF, Williams JG, Abelson HT, Green H, and Penman S: Cell 4: 69, 1975.
10. Johnson LF, Penman S, Green H: J Cell Physiol (in press).
11. Levis RW, Johnson LF, Abelson HT, et al: (in preparation).
12. Maaløe O, Kjeldgaard NO: Control of Macromolecular Synthesis: A Study of DNA, RNA, and Protein Synthesis in Bacteria. New York, W. A. Benjamin, 1966.
13. Mauck JC, Green H: Proc Natl Acad Sci USA 70: 2819, 1973.
14. Mauck JC, Green H: Cell 3: 171, 1974.
15. Mostafapour M-K, Green H: J Cell Physiol (in press).
16. Roeder RG, Chou S, Jaehning JA, Schwartz LB, et al: *In* Markert CL (ed): Isozymes III, Developmental Biology. New York, Academic Press, 1975, p 27–44.
17. Rudland PS: Proc Natl Acad Sci USA 71: 750, 1974.
18. Soeiro R, Amos H: Science 154: 662, 1966.
19. Stanners CP, Becker H: J Cell Physiol 77: 31, 1971.

Influence of Geometry on Growth of Normal and Malignant Cells

Judah Folkman, M.D.

In recent years it has become clear that nature uses an elaborate system of controls to assure that mammalian cells do not grow inappropriately. Most investigators have focused their attention on the humoral pathways responsible for many of these control points. Serum growth factors, growth inhibitors, and cell cyclic nucleotides are but a few. However, it has not been widely appreciated that geometrical configuration may also participate in growth regulation. The shape of an individual cell may permit, or prevent that cell from proliferating. The configuration of a population of cells may determine whether that population will remain dormant, or expand.

TUMOR CELL POPULATIONS

In Vivo. Our interest in the role of geometry in cell growth arose from studies of tumor angiogenesis, i.e., the capacity of growing tumors to induce the proliferation of new capillary blood vessels from the host [11,10]. We proposed that most solid tumors pass through two stages of growth: the *avascular* phase and the *vascular* phase (Fig. 1). During the early growth of a spontaneously arising tumor, a small nodule may reach a diameter of a few millimeters and a population in the range of 1 million cells. These tiny nodules survive in the tissues by simple diffusion of nutrients from the extravascular fluids. Further growth is possible only when new host blood vessels have penetrated into the tiny tumor, i.e., the onset of the *vascular phase*. If the hallmark of the avascular phase is growth restriction, then the principle feature of the *vascular* phase is rapid growth.

The distinction between these two phases is difficult to observe in experimental animals. By the time an inoculum of tumor cells has become barely palpable, it is already a vascularized tumor mass. The avascular phase is brief and imperceptible. To prolong the avascular phase for detailed study,

From the Department of Surgery, Children's Hospital Medical Center and Harvard Medical School, Boston, Mass.
Supported by USPHS Grant #RO1-CA14019.

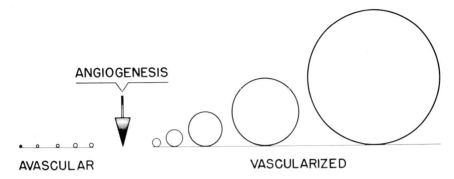

ANGIOGENESIS

AVASCULAR   VASCULARIZED

FIG. 1. The growth of most solid tumors can be separated into 2 stages. The avascular tumor is often an *in situ* carcinoma, and may be present for years without changing size. During the vascularized phase, rapid growth occurs. From Folkman [11].

we implanted tumors in the rabbit eye [15]. Brown-Pearce tumor cells were inoculated into the aqueous humor of the anterior chamber. Small spheroidal tumors appeared, but stopped growing at less than 1 mm diameter. They remained avascular as long as they were suspended in the aqueous humor, where new capillaries were unable to reach them. The spheroids remained viable as demonstrated by histology. Cells at the periphery of these spheroids incorporated ³H-thymidine, while cells in the center were necrotic. The spheroids remained viable indefinitely and could be transferred from one eye to another. However, they reached a steady-state in which cells being generated at the periphery were balanced by those dying in the center. Despite the nutrients which continually exchange around the spheroid due to the circulation of the aqueous humor, this form of three-dimensional growth was self-regulating. The tumor spheroids were measured daily with a stereoscopic slit-lamp. A maximum diameter was reached beyond which no further expansion occurred, until the spheroid was allowed to become vascularized. If the avascular spheroid was moved contiguous to the iris, new vessels penetrated the tumor and rapid growth followed (Fig. 2).

In Vitro. Is "population dormancy" of avascular spheroids unique to the eye, or is it a more general phenomenon? To answer this question, an *in vitro* counterpart of the avascular tumor was studied by suspending tumor cells in soft agar [12]. Single cells grew to small spheroidal colonies. Despite frequent renewal of the media, or transfer of the spheroids to fresh media, the final mean diameter of the spheroids was inversely proportional to the number of spheroids occupying the same flask (Fig. 3). With a moderate amount of crowding, spheroids stopped growing at 1 mm or less, just as in the anterior chamber. Could a single spheroid in a large flask of medium

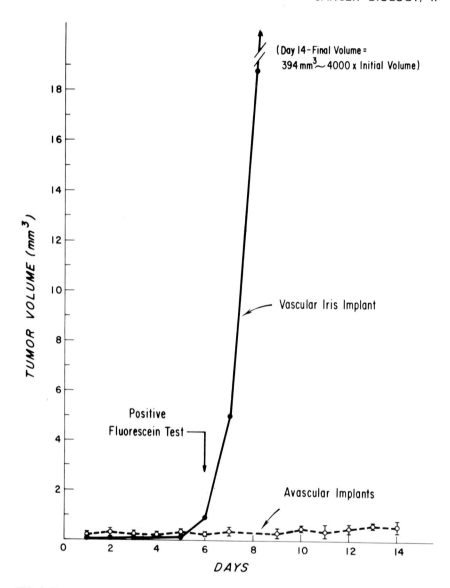

FIG. 2. The mean volumes of 10 avascular but viable spheroids of Brown-Pearce tumor floating in the anterior chamber, do not exceed 1 mm³. By contrast one of these spheroids which has been allowed to vascularize by being implanted on the iris. The vascularized tumor increased its volume by 16,000 times the initial volume of the avascular tumors. From Gimbrone et al. [15].

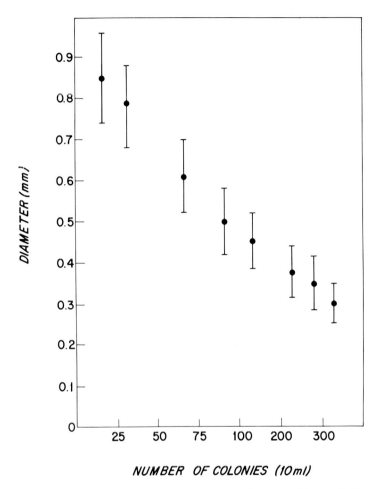

FIG. 3. When V-79 spheroids are crowded in the same flask, the "dormant" diameter is inversely proportional to the number of colonies. Other cell lines which grow as spheroids in suspension culture also behave this way.

escape this form of "dormancy"? No. Individual spheroids were removed to a fresh flask of media every other day. Such spheroids just arrived at the steady state with a slightly larger diameter. Population dormancy was achieved by 5–23 weeks, after which there was no further growth, for up to 40 weeks. The average diameter of the dormant stage for L-5178Y (mouse leukemia) cells was 3.8 mm ± 0.5 (Fig. 4). For B-16 mouse melanoma cells the dormant diameter was 2.4 ± 0.4 mm. Furthermore, spheroids of a given cell line each contained a limited number of viable cells. For example, the

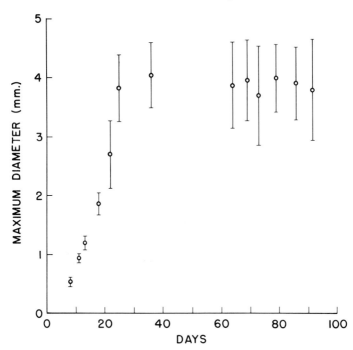

SPHEROIDS OF L5178y CELLS

FIG. 4. Mean diameter and standard deviations of 50 isolated spheroids of L-5178Y cells. Each spheroid was maintained alone in 10 ml soft agar and transferred every 2–3 days to a new flask. From Folkman and Hochberg [12].

maximum number of viable cells in the L-5178Y spheroids was approximately 3×10^5 (Fig. 5). Spheroids were exposed at various times to a single pulse of ^{3}H-thymidine and radioautographs were made. At less than 0.1 mm diameter, almost all cells were labeled. Beyond a diameter of 0.3 mm there was usually a central necrotic area, a middle zone of live but unlabeled cells, and an outer zone of labeled cells with accompanying mitoses. In spheroids up to 1.0 mm diameter, almost all cells on the surface, and 3–5 layers deep, were labeled with ^{3}H-thymidine (Fig. 6).

In the larger, dormant stage, the proliferative compartment of labeled cells occupied only one or two layers on the outermost rim of the spheroid. No matter how often the media was changed, and regardless of the amount of space available in each flask, all tumors stopped growing within the range of dormant size for a given tumor line. The only means of escape from this stringent growth limitation was a change in geometry of the cell population.

When the same population of cells was cultured in a *flat* configuration, growth was unlimited. The cell population expanded continuously, provided that media was exchanged frequently, and there was sufficient open space for cell growth. A working hypothesis to explain the difference between two-dimensional and three-dimensional cell population growth must take into account the surface area of the aggregate population [14]. For a flat culture growing only in two dimensions, surface area increases almost linearly with volume (Fig. 7). Therefore, surface area is always adequate for exchange of nutrients and wastes between the population of cells and its medium. By contrast, the surface area of a spheroidal population increases by the second power, as the volume increases by the third power (Fig. 8). In time, a population is reached where the surface area is inadequate to support all the cells by exchange of nutrients and wastes through simple diffusion. A steady state is achieved.

Another way to change the configuration of a spheroidal population of cells is to penetrate it with hollow fibers. Knazek [17] seeded transformed

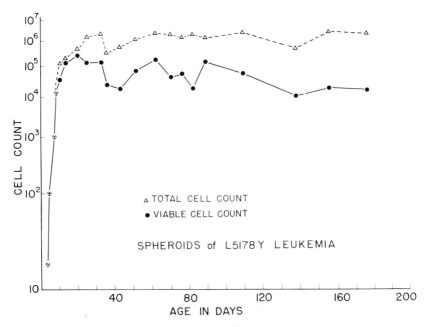

FIG. 5. Spheroids of L-5178Y depicted in Figure 4. The total cell number and the number of viable cells reach a steady state at approximately 30 days. From Folkman and Hochberg [12].

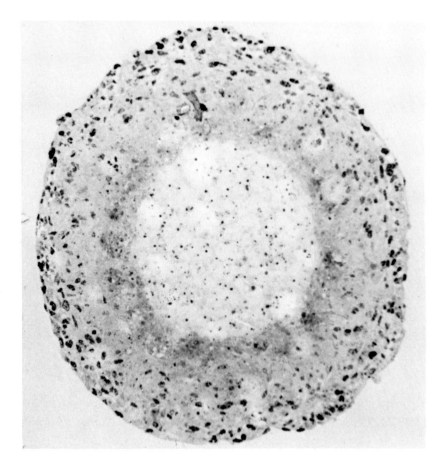

FIG. 6. H and E microsection of V-79 spheroid approximately 1.0 mm diameter and 20 days old. Five to seven outer cell layers are labeled with ^{3}H-thymidine. From Folkman and Hochberg [12].

cells among a group of semipermeable capillary tubes with a diameter of 200 microns. Tissue culture medium was perfused through the lumen of these fibers. In this arrangement, cells grew in a cylindric configuration; nutrients diffused into the colony from its center as well as its periphery. Cell densities around these capillary units were similar to those of solid tissue *in vivo*, i.e., approximately 10^8 cells/cc of tissue (Fig. 9).

Similarities between Geometrical Effects upon Tumors In Vivo *and* In Vitro. Malignant tumors *in vivo* may exist in four general types of configurations: (1) three-dimensional (i.e., spheroidal) without capillaries, (2)

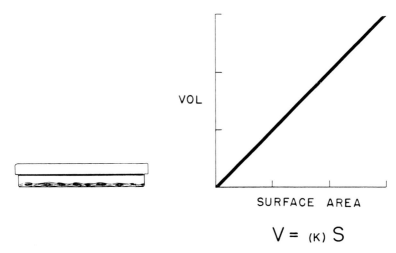

$$V = {}_{(K)} S$$

FIG. 7. The surface to volume relationship of a population of transformed cells growing in two dimensions. From Folkman et al. [14].

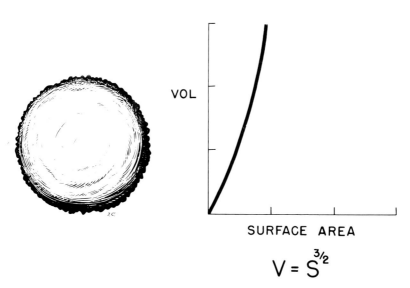

$$V = S^{3/2}$$

FIG. 8. The surface to volume relationship of a population of transformed cells growing in a three-dimensional configuration, i.e., as a spheroid. From Folkman et al. [14].

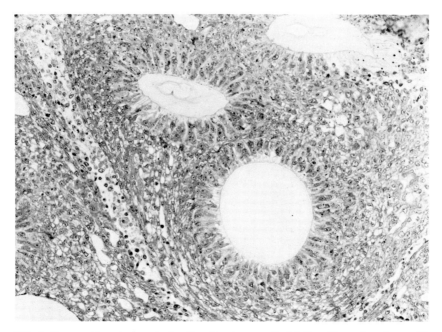

FIG. 9. Cross section micrograph of cells cultured on a unit of hollow fibers of semipermeable membrane. The unit is made up of polysulfone capillary tubes interspersed with silicone polycarbonate capillaries. The silicone tubes are permeable to gas and help to improve oxygen and carbon dioxide transport into the extracapillary space. The large cavities are lumens of artificial capillaries. The cells penetrate the crevices of the external wall, thus producing a columnar appearance around each capillary. Necrosis appears in cells distant from the capillaries. This section was made 4 weeks after inoculating 1×10^6 BT-20 cells from a monolayer culture. H&E $\times$ 138. Photograph courtesy of Dr. Richard Knazek [17].

three-dimensional with capillaries, (3) flat sheets or thin cords), and (4) ascites or bone marrow (similar to cell suspension).

The vast majority of early primary tumors, appear to choose the first two configurations. Carcinoma of the breast, colon, cervix, skin, bladder, liver etc. usually begins as a microscopic avascular nodule of tumor cells (i.e., the *in situ* tumor). This progresses to the vascularized tumor which has been penetrated by host capillaries. For some unknown reason, the capacity of a tumor to grow as a flat sheet, or as a thin cord of cells, along nerves and smooth surfaces (like pleura), develops very late, if ever. In human cancer, this capacity appears in the end stage of the disease after months or years of tumor "progression." The same is true for ascites formation. Although few solid tumors ever acquire the capacity to grow in the peritoneal fluid, those which do, develop this ability very late.

Therefore, the common pattern is for a small population of tumors cells (approximately 10^6) to survive in an avascular (*in situ*) nodule by simple diffusional exchange of nutrients and wastes with the surrounding tissue. This stage is limited for the same reasons that spheroids stop growing in soft agar. New capillaries which penetrate the avascular tumor provide an escape from the restrictions of a 3-dimensional, crowded population. The mechanism may be the same as the increased cell density which becomes possible *in vitro* when cells are cultured among semipermeable hollow fibers.

INDIVIDUAL NORMAL CELLS

In Vitro. The geometrical control over growth of neoplastic cells operates at the level of populations or groups of tumor cells. It is the shape of the *population* which permits or prevents continued growth. The shape of an individual tumor cell seems to have no effect upon its growth. By contrast, for the individual *normal* or nontransformed cell, shape is critical. For a normal cell, *cell shape* may determine whether it will proliferate or cease division; whether it will live or die. This phenomenon is nicely demonstrated in tissue culture. Diploid, untransformed fibroblasts, grown on plastic or glass, adhere and flatten out. They proliferate until confluence is reached. By contrast, when grown in suspension, either in soft agar, methyl cellulose, spinner culture or in static media over a nonadherent surface (such as agar), they fail to proliferate [18,20].

The major difference between the nongrowing cells and their proliferating counterparts is their shape. Cells in suspension become round or spheroidal, cells attached to plastic are flat and extended. Most normal or untransformed fibroblasts and epithelial cells cannot grow when suspended, and while they remain spherical. If kept in suspension they eventually die. Normal diploid cells, inhibited in suspension culture, can be rescued if they are allowed to stretch out on glass fibers or flatten out on glass beads, floated into the medium [20].

In Vivo. It is more difficult to discern whether the effect of "shape" on individual normal cells also operates in-vivo. Epithelial cells and fibroblasts are rarely found alone except during wound healing. Furthermore, some of these cells are stretched out on basement membranes; others are not. The majority are contacted on all sides by neighboring cells. However, there are at least two situations in-vivo which support the idea that flattening or extension of untransformed cells permits proliferation. One is tumor production by implantation of cells coated on glass beads. The other is foreign body carcinogenesis.

Implantation of Glass Beads: Balb/3T3 fibroblasts proliferate as a monolayer on plastic or glass *in vitro,* but will not grow in suspension culture. They do not form tumors when inoculated into histocompatible animals. However, if these cells are allowed to stretch out on glass beads (3 mm diameter) *before* implantation, tumors appear regularly, by about 8 weeks [3]. No tumors result from the implantation of beads alone, or cells alone. The new tumors are genetically stable and their daughter cells give rise to lethal tumors upon subsequent implantation in the absence of glass beads. This implies that the original 3T3 cells were not completely transformed, and not tumorigenic by themselves prior to the first implantation on glass beads. A period of further proliferation was apparently required to take the final step necessary to become a "successful" tumor. Attachment to the glass beads permitted this. The flat state seems to have been an essential feature contributing to the appearance of a clone of neoplastic cells.

Foreign Body Carcinogenesis: Implantation of a variety of smooth surfaces such as glass, plastic or steel into mice and rats will induce sarcomas [24,2,4]. For example, a coverslip of plastic or glass implanted subcutaneously will usually induce a sarcoma after approximately 9 months. Physical form is important; chemical composition is not. A variety of polymer sheets and films will produce tumors but powders of these materials will not. There is also a direct relationship between surface area and tumor incidence. Discs of less than 1 cm² are unlikely to induce a tumor while discs of 2 cm² or greater, are very carcinogenic [1]. Also the fibrous foreign body reaction which forms around an implant, is important, possibly as a source of cells which will eventually be involved in carcinogenesis. If the fibrous capsule is removed early, along with the implant, tumors usually do not develop. Tumors may develop if only the implant is removed late in the course.

Brand and his co-workers have carried out a series of experiments to understand etiology [22,5]. They used two CBA mouse strains differing only by a marker gene, T_6. A plastic disc was implanted subcutaneously. Clones of cells began to proliferate in the fibrous capsule and attached themselves to the plastic surface, where they continued to proliferate. When the disc was transferred to the mouse of different genetic makeup, the tumor which arose was always of the donor type (Fig. 10). This implies that the preneoplastic cells adherent to the plastic film were carried over to the recipient animal. Burnet [8] has proposed that the continuous proliferation which occurs on the plastic, may promote the selection of an intrinsic mutant which then accumulates as a clone of neoplastic cells. Whatever the origin

SMOOTH SURFACE CARCINOGENESIS

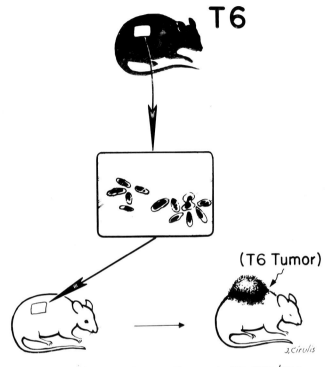

(K.G.Brand et al. Cancer Research 35:279,'75)

FIG. 10. Spindle shaped cells spread out and proliferate on a plastic film implanted into CBA/ H-T6 mouse. When the film is later transplanted to a CBA/H mouse, the tumor which develops is from the T6 donor. This is a diagrammatic summary of Brand's data [5].

of these cells, and by whatever path they become neoplastic, the analogy to flat tissue culture is striking. Normal diploid cells, allowed to proliferate continuously in monolayer cultures may eventually undergo spontaneous transformation. In fact, Brand and his co-workers [7] also found that cells which spread out on the implanted plastic discs, could be transferred to monolayer tissue culture, allowed to become preneoplastic or neoplastic *in vitro,* and reimplanted subcutaneously. The latent period before the appearance of tumors in recipients varied in relation to the number of passages *in vitro,* and also with the method of implantation. Cells from early culture passages, which were attached to plastic films at the time of implantation, reached neoplastic autonomy earlier than did the same cells inoculated into the animals as a suspension or pellet. This is reminiscent of 3T3 cells on glass beads. "Preneoplastic" cells which have not yet acquired all the characteristics necessary to produce a tumor when inoculated as free cells, can grow into a tumor when implanted while attached to a smooth surface.

Exposure to asbestos is another example of foreign body carcinogenesis. Asbestos fibers produce malignant mesotheliomas in man and in experimental animals. Asbestos fibers 20–320 microns long produced mesotheliomas when injected into the pleural cavities of rats [19]. Fibroblasts attached to the fibers and became extended. Proliferation followed. Fibers less than 20 microns did not cause mesotheliomas. These experiments suggest that from the standpoint of any given cell, it appears not to matter exactly how a "flat" configuration is achieved. Whether a fibroblast is spread out on a plastic film, or stretched out on a glass or asbestos fiber (i.e., extended), the result is the same; continuous proliferation.

THEORETICAL CONSIDERATIONS

The available evidence suggests that geometric control of growth operates at two levels; one for individual cells, the other for groups of cells, or cell populations. At each level, growth is halted unless the cell acquires some new property which allows it to escape and to resume growth.

For example, at the first level of geometric control, i.e., where individual normal cells are affected by their shape, a normal fibroblast is permitted to proliferate only when it is flat or extended. A variety of stimuli can initiate mitosis once the cell is in this required configuration. By contrast when it is spherical, such a cell is resistant to almost all mitotic stimuli. One route of escape is transformation (for example by an oncogenic virus). Transformed cells can proliferate regardless of their shape. They grow just as well when spherical (in suspension culture) as they do when flat (in monolayer culture).

However, even transformed cells are subject to a second type of geometric growth control, i.e., at the population level. At this level, an entire three-dimensional population of transformed cells may stop expanding because its surface to volume ratio becomes inadequate for diffusion of oxygen, nutrients and catabolites. The population becomes "dormant." A steady state is reached where the number of newly generated cells within the population equals the number of dying cells. Most transformed cells are unable to escape this form of growth control. A few can escape, because they have the capacity of inducing new capillaries to grow from the host and penetrate the tumor population. For convenience, these cells may be thought of as tumorigenic. The capacity to induce angiogenesis is one of the newly acquired properties which may allow a transformed cell to actually become tumorigenic. It may be profitable to examine this form of escape in more detail.

Tumor Angiogenesis: A Means of Escape from Population Dormancy. The ability of tumors to stimulate new capillary growth from the host appears to depend upon their secretion of a diffusible humoral factor, TAF [13], which is effective over distances of 2–5 millimeters [16]. Once host capillaries have penetrated a dormant tumor spheroid, its necrotic center disappears and rapid tumor growth (sometimes exponential growth) occurs. Experimental tumors have grown up to 16,000 times their initial volume within 2 weeks after they became vascularized [15]. By what possible mechanism could vascularization bring about such rapid and continuous growth?

A hypothetical diagram of tumor growth around a penetrating capillary can be assembled from available evidence (Fig. 11). Tumor cells tend to grow as cylindrical units surrounding a capillary [21,25]. Tannock and Steel [21] have also shown that viable tumor cells are found a mean distance of approximately 100 microns from the nearest open capillary. The oxygen diffusion distance for most tissues is in the range of 150 microns [23]. Our own studies suggest that the maximum rate of elongation for a capillary induced by tumor may be up to 0.8 mm/day [6]. A cylinder of tumor of 150 micron radius surrounding a capillary of 1.0 mm may contain up to 10^4 tumor cells. From a series of histologic sections of animal and human tumors, we can make a rough estimate that a capillary of 1 mm length will contain a minimum of 20 endothelial cells and a maximum of about 100 endothelial cells. Therefore, as the capillary elongates by the length of only one endothelial cell, approximately 100 new tumor cells can be supported. It is thus possible to perceive of neovascularization as an amplification step by which each new segment of capillary supplies the nutrients for a burst of new tumor growth.

In summary, geometric regulators of growth appear to act as gates. They give permission to proliferate or they withhold it. Of all the elaborate safeguards which protect against excessive mitosis, these may be among the most important.

How much can be said about the mechanism of each type of geometric control?

The second level of geometric control, i.e., the limitation of growth of three-dimensional cell populations, can be partly understood in terms of diffusion gradients and access of nutrient and catabolite molecules to crowded cell populations.

However, there is no satisfactory conceptual framework for the first level

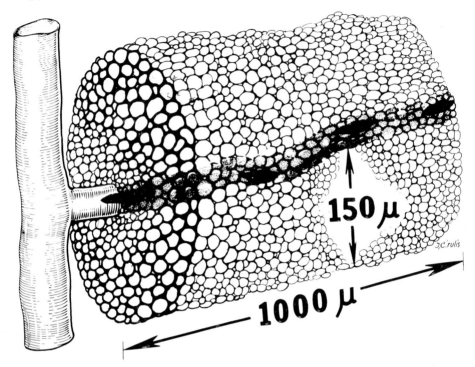

FIG. 11. Diagram of tumor cells as they might grow in a vascularized tumor. A cylindrical population of cells forms around the capillary. The capillary itself can grow from a relatively small
number of endothelial cells. Because the capillary supports a much larger population of tumor
cells, an amplification step exists. This amplification step may be responsible for the rapid
growth of a vascularized tumor.

of geometric control over *individual* normal cells. Why should flatness be so
healthy and so conducive to proliferation for a normal cell, while the
spherical shape leads to cessation of growth and eventual death? If flatness
is so important to the normal cell, what is the role of "anchorage
dependence"?

The concept of anchorage dependence introduced by Stoker and his
colleagues has been very helpful in describing an operational difference
between non-transformed and transformed cells. However, this term is difficult to translate into a possible perception of how DNA synthesis (and
perhaps also protein synthesis), might be linked to substrate attachment in
nontransformed cells. On a purely intuitive basis, it seems to me that "flatness" or "extension" may be more useful terms because it is conceivable
that a change in the geometry of the cell membrane, may in some way be
transmitted to the internal cell structures and thereby influence a variety

of synthetic mechanisms. Also, I have used "flatness" in preference to "anchorage dependence" in this monograph so that this state of the cell in culture could be compared to the spherical state.

At first glance, "anchorage" and "flatness" seem inextricably associated and it could be argued that substituting one word for the other is a fruitless exercise. But suppose that "flatness" is the critical requirement for normal cell growth in culture, and that "anchorage" is one way to achieve it, but not the only way. This problem cannot be adequately examined until some method is found to dissociate "anchorage" and "flatness." Or to put the problem another way, how would non-transformed cells behave if they could be flattened *without* "anchorage"? For example, we have recently found it feasible to grow cells by compression between parallel plates coated with materials to which these cells do not adhere, such as agar or cellulose acetate. At this writing, these experiments are too preliminary to say anything except that it is necessary to keep an open mind that flatness may be an essential requirement for proliferation and viability of nontransformed cells in culture.

Finally, it is possible that variations in surface tension over the cell membrane may turn out to play a role in the mechanism by which geometry influences cell growth. Surface tension phenomena are known to operate at the cellular level during cell culture. For example, the reason that a cell in suspension is forced to become spherical is the result of interfacial tension between the outer cell membrane and the surrounding medium. Furthermore, Carter's experiments [9] suggest that with substrates of decreasing surface tension, cells show decreasing adherence and are finally unable to flatten or spread out. It is entirely possible that changes in interfacial tension of the outer cell membrane which accompany changes in shape, may somehow be transmitted to internal cell structures such as microfilaments or microtubules in such a way as to influence protein synthesis or DNA synthesis. This, of course, is pure speculation and there is no information available at the moment which would permit deeper inquiry.

ACKNOWLEDGMENTS: The author appreciates the opportunity for the exchange of ideas and discussion with Drs. Harvey Greenspan and Sheldon Penman. I also thank Mr. Carl Cobb for editorial assistance and Mrs. Polly Breen for preparation of the manuscript.

REFERENCES

1. Alexander P, Horning ES: CIBA Foundation Symposium on Carcinogenesis. London, 1959, pp 24–26.
2. Bischoff F, Bryson G: Prog Exper Tumor Res 5: 85, 1964.
3. Boone CW: Science 188: 68, 1975.

4. Brand KG: *In* Becker FF (Ed): Cancer: A Comprehensive Treatise, Vol. I. New York, Plenum Press, 1975, pp 485–511.

5. Brand KG, Buoen LC, Johnson KH, Brank I: Cancer Res 35: 279, 1975.

6. Brem H, Folkman J: J Exp Med 141: 427, 1975.

7. Buoen LC, Brand I, Brand KG: J Natl Cancer Inst 55: 721, 1975.

8. Burnet M: *In* Intrinsic Mutagenesis: A Genetic Approach to Aging. New York, Wiley, 1974, pp 151–152.

9. Carter SB: Nature 210: 256, 1967.

10. Folkman J: Cancer Res 34: 2109, 1974.

11. Folkman J: *In* Klein G, Weinhouse S (Eds): Advances in Cancer Research, Vol. 19. New York, Academic Press, 1973, pp. 331–358.

12. Folkman J, Hochberg M: J Exp Med 138: 745, 1973.

13. Folkman J, Merler E, Abernathy C, Williams G: J Exp Med 133: 275, 1971.

14. Folkman J, Hochberg M, Knighton D: Cold Spring Harbor Symp. *In* Clarkson B, Baserga R (Eds): Cold Spring Harbor Conferences on Cell Proliferation, Vol. I, pp 833–842, 1974.

15. Gimbrone MA Jr, Leapman S, Cotran RS, Folkman J: J Exp Med 136: 261, 1972.

16. Gimbrone MA Jr, Cotran RS, Leapman SG, Folkman J: J Natl Cancer Inst 52: 413, 1974.

17. Knazek RA: Fed Proc 33: 1978, 1974.

18. MacPherson I, Montagnier L: Virology 23: 291, 1964.

19. Maroudas NG, O'Neill CH, Stanton MF: Lancet 1: 807, 1973.

20. Stoker M, O'Neill C, Berryman S, Waxman V: Int J Cancer 3: 683, 1968.

21. Tannock IF, Steel GG: J Natl Cancer Inst 42: 771, 1969.

22. Thomassen MJ, Buoen LC, Brand KG: J Natl Cancer Inst 54: 203, 1975.

23. Thomlinson RH, Gray LH: Br J Cancer 9: 539, 1955.

24. Turner FC: J Natl Cancer Inst 2: 81, 1941.

25. Wolter JR: J Ped Opthal 11: 62, 1974.

RNA Tumor Virus Genetics 1975

Peter K. Vogt, Ph.D.

The Genome of RNA Tumor Viruses

The genomic RNA of type C viruses is a single stranded linear molecule which sediments at 60 – 70 S and has a molecular weight of ∼6 – 10 × 10⁶ daltons. It consists of probably two hydrogen bonded components of approximately equal size which sediment, after dissociation by heat or dimethylsulfoxide, at about 35 S with an estimated molecular weight of 3 – 4 × 10⁶ daltons. Each of these 35 S components appears to contain all or almost all genes of the virus. The 70 S RNA is thus a polyploid structure comprising two identical or nearly identical nonsegmented unit genomes. Evidence for the polyploid, nonsegmented nature of the type C viral genome comes from transfection experiments with viral DNA and from studies on the biochemical complexity of the genome.

DNA extracted from avian sarcoma virus infected cells contains the genetic information of the virus and can infect new cells. The minimum molecular weight which is still compatible with infectivity of avian sarcoma virus DNA is 6 × 10⁶ daltons. Infection with this DNA follows single hit kinetics and suggests that the total information of the viral genome fits on a double stranded DNA of 6 × 10⁶ daltons. This figure corresponds to one 35 S component of RNA.

The complexity of viral RNA has been measured after digestion of the ³²P-labeled RNA with T-1 ribonuclease. From exhaustive digests oligonu-

From the Department of Microbiology, University of Southern California, School of Medicine, Los Angeles, Calif.

The author gratefully acknowledges the valuable contributions of Martin Alevy, Karen Beemon, Michael Bishop, Young Chen, Peter Duesberg, Michael Hayman, Eric Hunter, Michael Lai, Allan Tereba, Harold Varmus and Luhai Wang to the studies and ideas described above.

References to the recent genetics of RNA tumor viruses may be found in the Cold Spring Harbor Symposium 1975, in the Abstracts of the 1975 Cold Spring Harbor Tumor Virus Meeting and in the 1973, 1974 and 1975 volumes of Virology and the Proceedings of the National Academy of Sciences.

Work by the author is supported by Public Health Service Research Grant No. CA 13213 and by Virus Cancer Program Contract No. NOI CP 53518 awarded by the National Cancer Institute.

cleotides can be isolated by electrophoresis and homochromatography. The molecular weight, composition and partial sequence of these oligonucleotides have been determined, and the molecular complexity of the type C virus genome was calculated following the formula:

$$\frac{MW_{RNA}}{MW_{OLIG}} = \frac{CPM_{RNA}}{CPM_{OLIG}}$$

The data obtained by these technics in several laboratories are quite uniform and indicate that the complexity of genome is that of one 35 S RNA component and corresponds to a molecular weight of $3 - 4 \times 10^6$ daltons.

Most of the 35 S components contain poly-A at the 3′ end, and the T-1 oligonucleotide fingerprints of 35 S components without poly-A are identical to those with poly-A obtained from the same virus. The sequence of genes on the 35 S genome appears to be fixed rather than permuted as can be shown by mapping of the major oligonucleotides generated by T-1 ribonuclease. In such mapping experiments the RNA is fragmented by alkali into random size pieces ranging from 5 – 35 S. The molecules from the 3′ end of the genome can be obtained from these mixtures by the ability of poly-A to bind to Millipore filters or to poly-dT-cellulose and can then be fractionated according to size on sucrose density gradients. When individual ^{32}P-labeled fractions representing poly-A containing fragments of different lengths are digested with T-1 ribonuclease and fingerprinted, it is found that the complexity of the prints increases with the size of the poly-A containing fragment. Some oligonucleotides occur already in small fragments and therefore must be located close to the 3′ end of the genome, others can be found only in the larger fragments and are situated closer to the 5′ end of the genome. Certain of the oligonucleotides have been assigned to specific gene functions, and thus the fingerprinting of poly-A containing genome fragments allows the mapping of viral genes.

Genome Functions and Mutants

Conditional as well as nonconditional mutants of type C viruses have been isolated. The conditional mutants are temperature sensitive (ts). Many of the nonconditional mutants represent deletions. The mutants can be grouped into three classes according to their functional defects. Class T (also T⁻ or td for transformation defective) mutants lack transforming ability. Class R (also R⁻ or rd for replication defective) mutants cannot synthesize infectious progeny. Class C mutants have a defect in a viral gene required for transformation and replication alike. These classes of viral mutants represent the division of the viral genome into T, R and C functions.

T functions. Mutants of avian sarcoma viruses which are *ts* in the initiation and maintenance of transformation are relatively common. They are not complemented by wild type (*wt*) leukosis viruses nor by *td* deletion mutants derived from nondefective sarcoma viruses. These mutations must therefore be located within the *td* deletion which represents about 10 to 15% of the genome near the 3′ end. Although class T *ts* mutants were first thought to show complementation, suggesting the involvement of several viral genes in the T function, more recent studies have shown that the transformation seen after double infection with these *ts* mutants at the nonpermissive temperature is probably due to recombination, as the mutants replicate freely at this temperature and form *wt* recombinants. Thus the T function may be a single gene. There is indirect evidence that this gene acts through a transforming protein. Mutant infected cells which have been kept at the nonpermissive temperature become retransformed when shifted to permissive conditions. This retransformation can be prevented with cycloheximide and therefore may require the synthesis of a new functional transforming protein.

Besides the T function which controls initiation and maintenance of transformation (now referred to as T-1), there may exist another transformation-related function which is linked only to the initiation of the transformed state. This T-2 function reflects the activity of an early viral gene which operationally means that after an initial 12 hours at the permissive temperature a shift to the nonpermissive temperature fails to have a restrictive effect, because the transient *ts* phase of the infection has passed. *Vice versa* if the infection is started the nonpermissive temperature, viral induced transformation cannot be brought about after a shift to the permissive temperature at 12 hours postinfection or later. The puzzling property of the T-2 function is that it can be complemented by leukosis viruses or by *td* deletion mutants, and that class T-2 mutants can recombine with leukosis or *td* viruses to yield sarcoma virus which is *wt* in its transforming ability. Taken at face value, these observations would mean that leukosis or *td* viruses have retained an early function which is required in the induction of *sarcoma* transformation but is not needed for virus replication, because class T-2 mutants produce infectious progeny at the nonpermissive temperature. Alternatively one could imagine that the T-2 function is required for replication as well, but that replication is less sensitive to a defect in the T-2 gene. In this case T-2 would actually be a C function. This explanation is in line with the idea that *td* viruses do not retain genes which are not required for their replication.

R functions. Type C RNA tumor viruses contain about 7 major structural proteins which are likely to be coded for by the viral genome. Two of these proteins are glycosylated surface components. The others appear to form internal structures of the virion. The major nonglycosylated proteins are translated from a polycistronic message which yields a polyprotein precursor that is secondarily cleaved into functional structural proteins. The structural proteins of type C particles probably represent R functions of the genome. Most of them are not required for the maintenance of the transformed state, because various nonproducing transformed cell lines exist which lack one or the other of these structural proteins. Other R functions may be connected to the synthesis of virion progeny RNA. From the foregoing one could expect that genetic analysis would identify a large number of viral mutants which affect replication. However, so far only few class R mutants of type C viruses have been isolated and fewer have been studied thoroughly. Therefore, only isolated examples are available to illustrate R functions, and one will be discussed here.

Avian sarcoma virus *ts* mutant *LA*3342 carries a late mutation which prevents the synthesis of infectious virus. Operationally, this means that a shift to the nonpermissive temperature at any time after infection stops production of infectious virus. A shift to the permissive temperature allows a complete recovery of virus synthesis. By complementation and by recombination tests, *LA*3342 maps outside the two major deletions of avian sarcoma viruses, the *td* deletion representing the T-1 function and about 10 to 15% of the genome, and an *rd* deletion representing about 15 to 20% of the genome in the glycoprotein gene. *LA*3342 must therefore have *wt* T functions, which is expected; it must also produce *wt* glycoproteins. The latter conclusion is also supported by the fact at the nonpermissive temperature this mutant can induce cellular resistance to superinfection with another virus of the same glycoprotein specificity. This resistance indicates that a functional glycoprotein occupies receptors at the cell surface. As mentioned above, a downshift from the nonpermissive to the permissive temperature leads to a resurgence of virus synthesis in *LA*3342 infected cells. Virus titers reach control levels within ½ hour after the shift. This recovery of virus replication cannot be prevented by exposing the cells to cytosine arabinoside, actinomycin-D or cycloheximide immediately prior to the shift, which indicates that all viral components are made at the nonpermissive temperature: DNA provirus, viral RNA and viral proteins. Indeed, cells infected with *LA*3342 at the nonpermissive temperature release noninfectious viral particles. These products of infection are heavier than the infectious particles made at 35°, and they are more heterogeneous. Electron microscopic inspection reveals grossly aberrant structures budding from *LA*3342 infected cells at the nonpermissive temperature resulting in larger than normal particles. These particles lack a compact core and are often derived from multiple plasma membrane buds. In polyacrylamide electrophoresis the aberrant particles show all the major structural proteins found in infectious virions, but in addition they also contain four novel nonglycosylated proteins, referred to as mutant proteins. At least three of these four mutant proteins are viral, because they can be precipitated with appropriate antiviral serum. The appearance of these new nonglycosylated proteins which show immunologic cross reaction with structural components of infectious virions could be explained by a faulty cleavage of the polyprotein precursor from which the nonglycosylated proteins are derived. Pulse chase studies on the fate of this precursor have indeed uncovered a significant retardation of cleavage in mutant infected cells at the nonpermissive temperature. The data on *LA*3342 are thus in accord with the hypothesis that the mutation affects primarily the assembly of infectious virions, probably because at the nonpermissive temperature conformational changes in the polyprotein precursor interferes with the cleavage process on which the formation of functional structural protein depends. A mutant of murine leukemia virus which is similarly *ts* for a replication shows many features in common with *LA*3342.

R and T functions compared. By definition, R and T functions are nonoverlapping; one affects exclusively replication, the other transformation. This situation is also reflected by the structure of the RNA. Avian sarcoma viruses give rise to two major types of deletion mutants, *td* deletions which cannot transform and *rd* deletions which cannot replicate. A fingerprint analysis of T-1 ribonuclease digests derived from these deletion mutants demonstrates that there are specific oligonucleotides lost in the *td* deletions. These oligonucleotides most likely represent the T-1 function. In the *rd* deletion affecting the synthesis of glycoproteins other oligonucleotides have disappeared and thus may be linked to the glycoprotein function. The oligonucleotides which disappear in this *rd* deletion are different from those specific for the *td* deletion, providing evidence for the lack of overlap between R and T functions.

C functions. C functions are required for virus replication and cellular transformation. Viral genes controlling early processes of infection, notably RNA to DNA transcription and integration of the viral genome into cellular DNA, belong in this category. Examples for C functions are provided by the avian sarcoma virus *ts* mutants *LA*335 and *LA*337 which at the nonpermissive temperature can neither transform nor replicate and carry a thermolabile DNA polymerase. The temperature lability affects all three catalytic activities of the enzyme, RNA dependent DNA synthesis, DNA dependent DNA synthesis and RNase H activity, although the latter to a lesser degree.

In the avian type C viruses the virion DNA polymerase occurs in two molecular forms, the α-form with a molecular weight of ~60,000 daltons and the β-form with a molecular weight of ~100,000 daltons. It appears that α is derived from β; α contains the three enzymatic activities of the polymerase, and in LA335 and LA337 it also carries the temperature-sensitive lesion. As a result of the temperature-sensitive defect in the polymerase DNA synthesis in mutant infected cells at the nonpermissive temperature is reduced to less than 20% of the levels seen at the permissive temperature. The residual synthesis probably represents partial transcripts of viral RNA which may be started by the polymerase before its thermal inactivation but which are biologically nonfunctional.

Genetic experiments have provided a good correlation between biologic properties of LA335 and LA337 and the presence of a ts DNA polymerase. In recombination tests with wt leukosis virus, the temperature sensitivity in transformation and replication and in the enzyme are completely linked. Recombinants with the wt enzyme are also wt for focus formation and synthesis of progeny virus. Recombinants which have retained a ts polymerase are also ts in their biologic properties. Genetic revertants which have acquired the ability to synthesize viral progeny at 41° invariably contain wt enzymes.

In conclusion, the T, R and C functions of RNA tumor viruses are beginning to be characterized by conditional and nonconditional mutants. It appears that the T function is relatively simple, probably encompassing only one gene, whereas the R function must represent several viral genes, and the C functions may be complex as well.

Recombination

Recombination is common among RNA tumor viruses. It was first seen in double infections with nondefective avian sarcoma and avian leukosis virus having a different envelope specificity. In the mixed yields, recombinants can be identified which have acquired the glycoprotein envelope marker from the leukosis virus and the focus-forming ability from the sarcoma virus. All markers of RNA tumor viruses seem to be able to participate in genetic recombination. For instance, ts transformation markers can recombine with various envelope glycoprotein markers. Double infections with different ts mutants yield wt virus. Mutants which carry multiple ts mutations can recombine with wt leukosis or sarcoma virus to give single ts mutants. Not only does recombination occur between two viruses infecting the same cell from outside, but it also is found between exogenous virus and an endogenous virus integrated in the cell genome, provided that the endogenous virus is transcribed. An apparent exception to the generality of recombination between RNA tumor virus markers is provided by certain *rd* deletions such as the Bryan high titer strain of Rous sarcoma virus and possible murine sarcoma virus. These sarcoma viruses cannot recombine with a leukosis or leukemia virus to acquire their missing R functions. This defect in recombination is specific for the R functions which are located in the deletion, other viral genes of the Bryan high titer strain of Rous sarcoma virus and of similar *rd* deletions can participate in recombination. A possible explanation for this curious finding postulates that the T function of the deletion mutant occupies the genetic map position of the lost R function. Recombination may occur but would not be detectable, because it results in an exchange of nonallelic genes yielding recombinants which remain either *rd* or *td*.

The frequency of recombinants in mixed yields is unusually high, from 10 to 40%. This observation together with the fact that the 70 S RNA of the virion consists of two or more 35 S components first suggested that recombination between avian RNA tumor viruses may reflect reassortment of 35 S RNA segments. However, it is now known that 35 S RNA represents the entire genome of an RNA tumor virus, and thus there are no functionally specialized genome segments which could reassort. Therefore, recombinants must arise by molecular crossing over between homologous nucleic acid molecules. Three types of observation provide independent evidence for crossing over.

(i) In the cross between a nondefective avian sarcoma virus and an avian leukosis virus, the 35 S RNA of the two parental viruses shows a size difference of about 10 to 15%. Thus, 35 S RNA derived from either parent by reassortment would be recognizable, and recombinants having markers of the leukosis as well as of the sarcoma virus should contain large and small 35 S RNA. However, all sarcoma virus recombinants studied contain only the large RNA which suggests that crossing over has taken place.

(ii) When the RNA of recombinants is analyzed electrophoretically, minor size variations of approximately $\pm 70,000$ daltons are revealed. RNA derived from sarcoma virus recombinants which are selected for the same two markers but have originated from different recombinational events may be either slightly smaller or slightly larger than the RNA of the parental sarcoma virus. These size differences are characteristic of a given recombinant clone and are genetically stable. They cannot be explained on the basis of reassortment, but could arise from unequal crossing over which may lead to small deletions from the genome or add small duplications.

(iii) If we assume that the 70 S complex consists of maximally three 35 S components, then reassortment of these components can lead to only two different combinations. The two 35 S components carrying the selected markers must be the same in both combinations. The third 35 S component which is not affected by the selection may be derived from either parent and would provide the only source of variability in genetic sequence. However, fingerprint patterns of recombinant RNA prepared after T-1 ribonuclease digestion have shown a much greater diversity of sequences. In two crosses the first five recombinant clones investigated all showed different finger-prints. This result can be explained by crossing over, because the position of the crossover point would vary with different recombinants. The sequence diversity would also be increased by multiple cross overs and by crossovers outside the markers tested.

High frequency crossover between single stranded RNA molecules has not been observed in other systems and therefore other mechanisms must be considered for crossing over between RNA tumor viruses. An acceptable hypothesis proposes that in the first round of double infection heterozygotes are formed which is a likely event because of the polyploidy of the 70 S genome. These heterozygotes would be the precursors of recombinants. Recombination could occur in the second round of infection during RNA-DNA transcription of heterozygotes. Under these circumstances the two parental genomes are enclosed and the same virus particles and united in the same 70 S complex. This proximity may greatly enhance genetic exchange. In favor of this hypothesis it may be noted that heterozygotes are indeed found in double infections with RNA tumor viruses. Furthermore, recombination between RNA tumor viruses has been shown to require more than one cycle of infection as would be expected if heterozygotes were the obligatory precursors of recombinants. The fact that integrated virus DNA which is not transcribed fails to participate in recombination is also in accord with this hypothesis. A detailed understanding of the mechanism by which RNA tumor viruses recombine will be necessary for genetic mapping experiments, and in turn the outcome of mapping tests will reflect on the mechanism of recombination.

Future work on the genetics of RNA tumor viruses will no doubt make increasing use of newly developed technologies in nucleic acid chemistry. Fingerprinting of mutant RNAs, sequencing of the RNA and locating specific oligonucleotides along the genome, as well as analysis of the DNA transcripts with restriction endonucleases, all promise rapid advances in this area, especially if complemented by the more traditional genetic approaches of mutant isolation and characterization.

BACKGROUND READING

Beemon K, Duesberg PH, Vogt PK: Proc Natl Acad Sci USA 71: 4254, 1974.

Duesberg PH: Proc Natl Acad Sci USA 60: 1511, 1968.

Duesberg PH, Vogt PK: Proc Natl Acad Sci USA 67: 1673, 1970.

Duesberg PH, Vogt PK: Virology 54: 207, 1973.

Vogt PK: Virology 46: 939, 1971.

Vogt PK: Virology 46: 947, 1971.

Vogt PK: Possible episomes in eukaryotes. *In* Silvestri L (Ed): Proc Fourth Lepetit Colloquium. Amsterdam, North Holland Publishing Co., 1973.

Weiss RA, Mason WS, Vogt PK: Virology 52: 535, 1973.

Type C Virogenes: Genetic Transfer and Interspecies Transfer

G. J. Todaro, M.D.

Transmission of Virogenes

In the course of studies on the development of mouse cell lines in culture [2,14] it was noted that certain spontaneously transformed cells began to release type C RNA tumor viruses [1]. This finding, along with several observations from Dr. Robert Huebner's laboratory on the presence of viral specific antigens in the embryo of several mouse strains, led to the hypothesis (virogen-oncogene hypothesis) [7,15] that the information for the formation of such viruses might be transmitted genetically from parent to progeny along with other cellular genes (Table 1).

Activation of this normally repressed genetically transmitted type C virogene information, rather than infection from outside the animal, was proposed as the most common mechanism by which type C RNA tumor viruses are maintained in animal populations and produce naturally occurring cancers. Much subsequent experimental work supports this, the most important being that "virus-free" cell lines (Table 2) derived from chicken, mouse, hamster, rat, pig, cat and baboon tissues can begin to secrete, either spontaneously or after treatment with chemical inducing agents, typical complete type C viruses, Cocultivation with permissive cell lines from heterologous species has been needed to detect and to amplify virus production in several instances. In general, avian and mammalian cells in culture have been resistant to superinfection by their own endogenous type C viruses. The properties which characterize such endogenous mammalian type C viruses, the products of the genetically transmitted virogenes, are summarized in Table 3.

The endogenous type C virogenes are those sets of gene sequences coding for the production of type C viruses that are an integral part of the host species' chromosomal DNA. These genetically transmitted endogenous virogenes should be distinguished from type C viral DNA sequences which can be added to the animal's genome by "exogenous" viral infection and subsequent integration (provirus formation) [11]. Endogenous type C

From the Viral Leukemia and Lymphoma Branch, National Cancer Institute, Bethesda, Md.

TABLE 1. Implications of the Virogene-Oncogene Hypothesis

Virogenes
1. All somatic cells of a species have DNA homologous to type C virus RNA of that species (virogenes).
2. Type C viruses derived from closely related species should have closely related specific antigens, e.g., gs antigens, polymerase and their nucleic acid sequences should be more related to one another than are those viruses released by distantly related species (virogene evolution).

Oncogenes
3. The transformation specific sequences of RNA tumor viruses should be present in normal cellular DNA (oncogenes).
4. Spontaneous, chemically induced and viral induced transformed cells and tumor cells should have RNA as well as DNA sequences homologous to the transforming specific sequences found in tumor viruses (oncogene expression).

---

virogenes should also be distinguished from those gene sequences not originally present in the genome, that are postulated to form by gene duplication and/or recombination during the lifetime of the animal through the mediation of the reverse transcriptase [3,13] mechanism (protovirus formation) [12] (Table 4).

The sets of virogenes that a particular species possesses are normally repressed, but can be activated by a variety of intrinsic (genetic, hormonal) as well as extrinsic (radiation, chemical carcinogens, other infecting viruses) factors. As cellular genes, type C virogenes are subject to the pressures of mutation and selection; as such, closely related animal species would be expected to have closely related endogenous type C virogenes. *What is unique about type C virogenes as distinguished from most other cellular genes, however, is that, at least in some species, they can give rise to the production of infectious type C virus particles.*

Since endogenous type C virogenes code for the production of particles

TABLE 2. Species where a Complete Virogene Is Known to be Present in Normal Cells

---

Chicken	Rat
Chinese Hamster	Cat
Syrian Hamster	Pig
Mouse (*Mus musculus*)	Baboon
Mouse (*Mus caroli*)	

TABLE 3. Properties of Endogenous Type C Virogenes

1. In the DNA of all somatic and germ cells of all the animals in a species.
2. Multiple related but not identical copies present in the cellular DNA, more than DNA from a heterologous cell that is actively producing virus.
3. Virus expression (RNA, gs antigen, polymerase, complete particles) under cellular control. Expressed in certain tissues at certain times during development.
4. Cells generally resistant to exogenous infection by the homologous endogenous virus.
5. Clonal lines either spontaneously or after induction are capable of releasing complete virion.

secreted by the cell and contain specific viral proteins, a reverse transcriptase, and a high molecular weight RNA, their study appears to offer unique possibilities for purifying a discrete set of cellular genes and their products.

Isolation of Endogenous Primate Type C Viruses

Six separate isolates of infectious baboon type C virus have been obtained in this laboratory by cocultivation of kidney, lung, testes and placenta from several different species of baboon (*Papio hamadyas* and *Papio cynocephalus*), using suitable permissive host cell lines. These isolates are all morphologically and biochemically typical of mammalian type C viruses, but

TABLE 4. Major Differences between Virogene and Protovirus Models

Virogene	*Protovirus*
1. Complete copies present in germ cells and somatic cells.	1. Germ cells lack virus information. Generated in rare somatic cells by chance.
2. Genes maintained in population by normal cellular replication. Reverse transcriptase *not required*.	2. Reverse transcriptase plays essential role in generating new viruses.
3. Transformation results from activation of normally latent cellular genes associated with and/or part of the viral gene sequences.	3. Transformation results from the generation of new gene sequences by reverse transcription that do not pre-exist.

are distinctly different by immunologic and nucleic acid hybridization technics from all other previously studied type C viruses [4,16]. Further, the six isolates are all highly related to each other by host range, viral neutralization and interference, and by immunologic and nucleic acid hybridization criteria. ^{3}H-DNA transcripts prepared from three of the baboon type C virus isolated hybridize completely to DNA extracted from various tissues of several different healthy baboons. Such data suggested that these type C virus isolates were, indeed, endogenous viruses of baboons.

If the baboon type C viruses were truly endogenous primate viruses and had evolved, then it appeared reasonable to suspect that other Old World monkeys that are close relatives to the baboon would have related virogene sequences in their DNA. Those primate species less related to baboons taxonomically would be expected to have much more extensive mismatching of their virogene sequences.

The prosimians evolved from primitive mammalian stock roughly 60 to 80 million years ago. The New World monkey branch diverged from the common stem, leading to both the apes and the Old World monkeys approximately 50 million years ago. The Old World monkeys (which include the baboon species) have been separated from the great apes and from man for 30 to 40 million years.

Hybridization studies employing an endogenous baboon type C viral (^{3}H) DNA probe were used to detect type C viral nucleic acid sequences in primate cellular DNA. *Sequences related to those of the baboon type C virus are found in all other Old World monkey species, higher apes, and, of particular importance, they are also found in man.* The results presented support the conclusion that, within the primates, type C viral genes have evolved as the species have evolved, with virogenes from more closely related genera and families showing more sequence homology than those from distantly related taxons. The ubiquitous presence of endogenous type C virogenes among anthropoid primates and their evolutionary preservation for at least 30 to 40 million years suggest that such genes provide functions with a selective advantage to the species possessing them. They clearly have evolved in primates over the past 30–40 million years as stable cellular elements [5].

Transmission of Type C Genes between Distantly Related Species

The endogenous type C viruses of baboons and domestic cats are related, but can be distinguished, by biologic and immunologic criteria and by partial nucleic acid sequence homology. Virogene sequences in the DNA of

TABLE 5. Relationship between Cat and Baboon Endogenous Type C Virus

1. The cat (RD-114/CCC) and baboon virus groups are *related but distinct* from one another by:
   a. viral DNA-RNA hybridization,
   b. inhibition of polymerase activity by antibody,
   c. antigenicity of the p30 protein,
   d. viral interference,
   e. viral neutralization.
2. Cat and baboon unique sequence DNA markedly different; species diverged from one another over 80 million years ago.
3. Cat (RD-114/CCC) virus DNA transcripts hybridize to the DNAs of *all* Old World monkeys and apes, and to the DNAs of domestic cats and certain other felis species.
4. Baboon (M/M28) virus DNA transcripts hybridize to the DNAs of all Old World monkeys, higher apes, and man, and to DNAs of those felis species which contain RD-114 related sequences.

Old World monkeys and domestic cats also show a degree of relatedness not shared by the unique sequence DNA of these species. Genes related to the nucleic acid of an endogenous domestic cat type C virus (RD-114) are found in the cellular DNA of anthropoid primates while many members of the cat family *Felidae* lack these sequences (Table 5). Endogenous viruses from one group of mammals (primates) are thus concluded to have infected and become part of the germ line of an evolutionarily distant group of animals, ancestors of the domestic cat [6]. The data demonstrate that *viral genes from one group of animals can give rise to infectious particles that not only can integrate into the DNA of animals of another species, but can also be incorporated into the germ line (germ line inheritence of acquired virus genes)*. Clearly, if viral gene sequences can be acquired in this way it is possible that type C viruses have served to introduce other genes from one species to another, and may provide an important mechanism by which species stably acquire new genetic information.

Detection of Endogenous Type C Viral Gene Products in Primates Including Man

Competitive radioimmunoassays which detect the major viral structural protein (p30) of baboon type C viruses also detect viral antigen in certain normal baboon tissues, in a normal stumptain macaque spleen and a rhesus ovarian carcinoma. The p30 antigen from these tissues is closely related by several immunologic criteria to the p30 antigen from these tissues is closely related by several immunologic criteria to the p30 protein of baboon type C viruses. The results indicate that normal primate tissues translate at least one viral structural protein [9].

Partially purified extracts from 33 human tumors of several histologic types were used as competing antigens in a radioimmunoassay for the p30 protein of endogenous baboon type C virus. Antigens immunologically related to the p30 protein of the M7 baboon virus were detected in two tumors (a lymphoid lymphoma and an ovarian carcinoma). Like viral p30 antigens previously identified in tissues of several other primates, the antigens found in human tumors cross-react with the p30 protein of the RD-114 virus but are unrelated by similar immunologic criteria to the p30 proteins of several other mammalian type C viruses. Gel filtration shows that most of the antigenic activity cochromatographs with authentic p30 protein. These results, along with those showing nucleic acid sequences related to those o: an endogenous primate type C virus in the DNA of human cells, make it clear that humans, like other primates, have type C viral sequences in their genome and can, in some circumstances, express at least one type C viral protein [10].

The Possible Role of Viruses as Natural Transmittors of Genes between Species

In recent months considerable interest has been focused on the possibilities and risks associated with the introduction of new genes into the germ line of a species. Genes can be inserted into or deleted from bacterial viruses in the laboratory by simple chemical manipulation. But what is known about the natural role of viruses as transmittors of genes in higher organisms?

In our laboratory in the past year we have developed evidence, as described above, that shows that RNA tumor virus (type C virus) genes have been maintained as stable endogenous genetic elements in primates, including man, for at least 30–40 million years. Viruses from an ancestor of the modern Old World monkeys also could be shown to have entered the germ line of ancestors of the domestic cat (Table 6). From the relatives of the domestic cat that have this virus and from those that did not acquire it, we have concluded that the infection occurred 3–10 million years ago somewhere in Africa or in the Mediterranean Basin region. Because of the stability of the viral gene sequences when they are incorporated into cellular DNA, events that have occurred millions of years ago still can be

Table 6. Examples of Transmission of Type C Virus Genes between Species

Donor	Recipient	Genetically Transmitted in Recipient
Primate (Old World Monkey)	Felis (Ancestor of the domestic cat)	Yes
Rodent (Mouse Ancestor)	Pig Ancestor	Yes
Rodent (Asian Mouse, *M. caroli*)	Primates and Humans	No

recognized by examining the genetic information of the virus and that of the host cell.

More recently, our laboratory has found a second example of gene transmission between species, in this case from an ancestor of the mouse to an ancestor of the domestic pig. Pig cell cultures produce type C viruses that can be shown to be genetically transmitted and present in all pig tissues in multiple copies in the cellular DNA. Close relatives, such as the European wild boar and the African bush pig, have closely related viral genes in their DNA. It can be shown that this virus was acquired by an ancestor of the pig from a small rodent related to the mouse.

The genetically transmitted type C virus of the Asian mouse species, *Mus caroli,* can be shown to be closely related to the cancer-producing infectious primate type C viruses from gibbons, woolly monkeys and, perhaps, humans [8].

That viruses can transmit themselves between the DNA of very different species has been established as a result of experiments in our own laboratory in the past year. That they can carry cellular gene sequences from cell to cell also has been clearly demonstrated. That this transmission of cellular gene information *between species* has been a major force in evolution remains a speculation without, at the moment, any direct proof.

Viruses are unique in that they can serve to carry information between genetically isolated species. Classic Darwinian evolution deals with changes that occur by mutation and selection, duplication and rearrangement; the genetic information of a species can be changed and rearranged, but not added to from the outside. Viruses, such as the RNA tumor viruses, offer the possibility of additions of new gene sequences to a species. The type C

TABLE 7. Possible Functions of Genetically Transmitted Virogenes in Normal Cells

1. Activation of oncogenic information, while inappropriate in adult tissue, plays a normal role during differentiation and development.
2. The integrated virus serves to protect the species against related, more virulent infectious type C viruses.
3. Virus activation, being linked to transformation, protects the animal by altering the cell membrane. The released virus could alert the immune system making the transformed cells more susceptible to immunologic control.
4. As conveyors of genetic information between species they may have had an evolutionary role. Only this group of viruses has been shown to transmit genes between germ cells of different species under natural conditions.

viruses as a group, are uniquely suited for this role since they must incorporate into the cellular DNA in order to replicate and they also do not kill the cells they infect. Each time they move from cell to cell they have the possibility of carrying with them host cell genes. They thus provide a means of communication between cells of different species and different phyla; they serve to keep a species in communication with its neighbors-ecologic neighbors as well as genetic neighbors. Some of the possible normal functions that the virogene system may be involved in are summarized in Table 7.

Of course these same genes can transmit information that may disrupt normal cellular control and, by so doing, lead to the development of cancer in the individual. The cases of genetic significance, however, are when the new genes are incorporated into the germ line. The ease with which type C viruses can pick up host genes and can cross species barriers along with the general lack of lethal effect of these viruses makes them ideally suited for this kind of role.

Laboratory created viruses might facilitate the incorporation of genes of particular interest, but clearly viruses have had that capability long before modern man appeared on the earth. Mammalian germ-cells, then, our experiments show, are susceptible to viral-mediated acquisition of new genetic information.

REFERENCES

1. Aaronson S, Hartley J, Todaro GJ: Proc Natl Acad Sci USA 64: 87, 1969.
2. Aaronson S, Todaro GJ: Science 162: 1024, 1968.
3. Baltimore D: Nature 226: 1209, 1970.

4. Benveniste RE, Lieber MM, Livingston DM, et al: Nature 248: 17, 1974.
5. Benveniste RE, Todaro GJ: Proc Natl Acad Sci USA 71: 4513, 1974.
6. Benveniste RE, Todaro GJ: Nature 252: 456, 1974.
7. Huebner R, Todaro GJ: Proc Natl Acad Sci USA. 64: 1087, 1969.
8. Lieber MM, Sherr CJ, Todaro GJ, et al: Proc Natl Acad Sci USA 72: 2315, 1975.
9. Sherr CJ, Benveniste RE, Todaro GJ: Proc Natl Acad Sci USA 71: 3721, 1974.
10. Sherr CJ, Todaro GJ: Proc Natl Acad Sci USA. 71: 4703, 1974.
11. Temin HM: Ann Rev Microbiol 25: 609, 1971.
12. Temin HM: Proc Natl Acad Sci USA 69: 1016, 1972.
13. Temin HM, Mizutani S: Nature 226: 1211, 1970.
14. Todaro G, Green H: J Cell Biol 17: 299, 1963.
15. Todaro GJ, Huebner RJ: Proc Natl Acad Sci USA 69: 1009, 1972.
16. Todaro GJ, Sherr CJ, Benveniste RE, et al: Melnick JL: Cell 2: 55, 1974.

Type-C Viruses and Leukemia

Robert C. Gallo, M.D.

Type-C RNA tumor viruses (oncornaviruses) have been isolated from numerous species. Since the pioneering work of Ludwig Gross, they have been implicated as one major cause of leukemia [28]. The evidence for this varies substantially in different species. In some, we have only association of virus with the disease. In others, there is not only association but also ability of the investigator to reproduce the disease in another animal, sometimes of the same species but other times only in a heterologous host. Finally, in a few species there is virtually conclusive evidence that the virus is the cause of the disease. Here the evidence includes not only association and ability to reproduce the disease but also some additional data such as clear seroepidemiologic results. Examples of these include feline, bovine, and at least some primate leukemias. Generally speaking, the evidence is clear when the virus causes the disease as an infectious agent, horizontally transmitted. When transmission is more complex, such as in congenital infection (the probable cause of most viral leukemia in chickens [61]), it is much more difficult to conclusively show that the virus is the causative agent. There are important lessons to be learned from the experiences with feline and bovine leukemia, especially the former, but since these topics have recently been reviewed by experts in these particular fields [11], I will not discuss them here. Suffice it that just a few years ago epidemiologists argued that there was no evidence to indicate that these were infectious diseases. We now know that they are.

Particular Problems Complicating Proof that Type-C Viruses Cause Leukemia

There are a number of factors that make it difficult to prove these virus are the cause of natural leukemia, particularly in some species. *First,* even when they apparently cause disease as an infectious agent transmitted from animal to animal, there is generally a very long latency period. Therefore,

From the Laboratory of Tumor Cell Biology, National Cancer Institute, Bethesda, Md.

epidemiology is often complicated. *Second,* type-C viruses may be transmitted congenitally [2], and they also can be transmitted vertically in the form of the integrated DNA provirus (see below). In these instances, activation of the virus may occur randomly, induced perhaps by an environmental event. Clearly, in these instances there may be no epidemiologic pattern. *Third,* various type-C viruses have different properties. Some do not appear to be pathogenic for their natural host, and might even be involved in normal functions (see below). Identification of these viruses may complicate the picture when looking for a leukemogenic type-C virus. *Fourth,* to fulfill Koch's postulates in man is, of course, impossible, but even in animals it may not in the strict sense be possible. There is evidence that a virus isolated from a cell contains genetic differences from the virus which infected the cell. Presumably, this develops as a consequence of recombination of the provirus with host DNA. Both cell and virus can be genetically modified [24].

Replication of Type-C Viruses

A considerable amount of information on the biochemistry of type-C virus replication is now available. The recently published Cold Spring Harbor Volumes on Tumor Viruses (1975, Vol 39) contain numerous papers giving the latest information from most laboratories. In addition, there are at least 2 recent reviews [25,27]. Therefore, I will only briefly discuss the salient features of virus replication. (1) On infection, the virus adheres, penetrates, and uncoats. Little is known about these mechanisms. The use of viral pseudotypes has contributed to our understanding of the host range [61]. (2) Early after infection, within a few hours, the DNA provirus is synthesized from the viral RNA genome. This reaction is catalyzed by the virion specific DNA polymerase, reverse transcriptase. Work by Dahlberg and associates indicates that a specific tRNA (tryptophan tRNA for avian viruses) is the initiator (primer) nucleic acid *in vitro* [9]. The newly synthesized DNA is covalently attached to the $3'$-OH end of the primer and hydrogen bonded to the viral RNA template. This tRNA is a cellular species apparently incorporated into the virus. It will be important to determine if this is, in fact, the physiologic primer, i.e., to identify this as the primer in intact cells. As yet no one has identified the primer *in vivo.* (3) After formation of this RNA · DNA hybrid, the next steps are not yet completely clear. These viruses also contain a nuclease, RNase H, which specifically hydrolyzes an RNA moiety of a matched RNA · DNA hybrid. Some believe this is the next event in the virus replication cycle accompanied by synthesis of the DNA^+ strand. The double stranded DNA may then integrate into the host after circularizing (see H. Varmus, M. Bishop, and colleagues, Cold Spring Harbor Vol. 39 on Tumor Viruses). Others believe the hybrid itself integrates. It is possible that both processes occur. We do not know if all provirus synthesized integrates. (4) After integration the provirus may remain dormant or be partially or fully expressed. Little is known about the control mechanisms involved. What is known is that different proviruses can be under different control mechanisms. There is no evidence for any novel RNA polymerase. Transcription of the DNA provirus to viral RNA probably involves a host RNA polymerase. Probably after transcription poly A is added. The function of the poly A is not known but may add stability to the RNA (G. Marbaix, personal communication). (5) Translation of the viral RNA to viral specific proteins is the subject of investigation in many laboratories. It appears that large precursor proteins are first synthesized which are then cleaved to form the mature proteins. How many proteins are coded for by the viral genome is not known. It is clear that reverse transcriptase is viral coded and the data indicates that the p30 and gp 69–70 proteins are also probably viral coded. It is likely that other viral structural proteins are also viral coded. (6) Assembly and release or the last stages in the virus replication cycle are perhaps the least understood. There are observations which indicate that glucocorticoids are involved in the regulation of these processes.

Origin and Genetic Modification of Type-C Viruses

RNA tumor viruses grouped together from many species can be put into two classes. Class I are those which appear to be endogenous to the cell. Most have not been shown to be tumorigenic. We believe they may play a normal physiologic role in development. Support for this comes from observations that they are expressed more frequently in embryonic life and more directly from recent experiments in mice which indicates that one of the endogenous type-C viral proteins may be the same as the G IX protein of the developing thymus gland [32]. Molecular hybridization of the RNA genome of these viruses to DNA from the normal host cells indicates that most if not all of their sequences can be found in DNA from normal cells of the host species. These viruses can often be isolated from normal tissues, even those obtained from adult animals. Often they are detected (and subsequently isolated) after chemical induction, e.g., after treatment with iododeoxyuridine [59]. In the absence of whole virus particles, components of these viruses (RNA and/or proteins) are often found in normal embryonic tissues [38]. New isolates (not yet manipulated in the laboratory) aften are unable to replicate in cells obtained from their species of origin, but

PROPOSED MECHANISM FOR FORMATION OF
CLASS II ONCOGENIC RNA VIRUSES

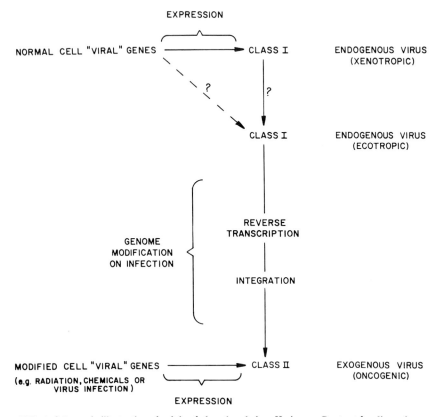

FIG. 1. Schematic illustration of origin of class 1 and class II viruses. See text for discussion.

they do infect heterologous cells. These are called endogenous xenotropic type-C viruses [33]. Other class 1 type-C viruses do replicate in cells of their homologous host. These are called ecotropic [33]. We believe that the xenotropic type-C viruses may be precursors of the ecotropic viruses (see Fig. 1). The data taken together indicate that the class 1 viruses had their origin in the genes of normal cells. An alternative possibility is that they originated independently, infected the germ line, and over a long period evolved toward the cell. In any case, the available information strongly implies that the class 1 "viral" genes and cell genes evolved together over a substantial period of time [59]. A molecular mechanism for the origin of the RNA genome of these viruses has been recently presented elsewhere [25].

The second class of RNA tumor viruses (class 2) contain an RNA genome which contains nucleotide sequences which are detectably different from the DNA of the normal host cell. Most of these viruses are oncogenic in laboratory experiments. We have proposed that these viruses originated by evolution of a class 1 RNA genome through one of two routes. The first of these is the modification of the viral genome which occurs after infection of new cells [24]. Thus, a class 1 viral RNA may evolve away from the parent cellular DNA under natural conditions when the virus is horizontally transmitted (animal to animal). The greatest genetic change may occur on infection of a different species.

In the laboratory, the investigator can enhance the evolutionary change by deliberating and repeatedly infecting cells, and evidence for change in viral RNA on infection has been described. The change in the viral genome on infection could be a consequence of infidelity of reverse transcriptase, i.e., an unfaithful transcript of the viral RNA may be synthesized [4]. Alternatively, and more likely, changes in the viral genome probably occurs during the recombination process of the newly synthesized proviral DNA and host cell DNA. We have found that after infection in some cases portions of the infecting viral genome is lost and new information from the infected cell may be acquired [25]. Similar observations were made earlier by Scolnick et al. [48]. Surprisingly, the major viral proteins are clearly conserved even after repeated infection of many heterologous cells. In this scheme it is also possible that if a class 1 (or class 2) virus of one species infects a new species and becomes stably associated with the new species, it will become a class 1 virus of the new species. This is, in fact, the interpretation Todaro and associates have made for the origin of the RD114 class 1 virus of cats from a primate virus [59].

The second possible route for creation of a class 2 type-C virus genome may be by direct modification of the class 1 "viral" genes in the cell, e.g., by radiation, chemical mutation, or by interaction with infecting viruses. (This, in effect, proposes that the class 1 viral genes include "hot spots", the virogene-hot spot theory, and has been discussed elsewhere [16].) Modified class 1 genes if completely expressed (DNA RNA) could then lead to the formation of a type-C virus with nucleotide sequences which have been altered, i.e., different from normal host cell and hence the progenitor of a class 2 virus. We have proposed that class 1 genes are important to normal differentiation, and modification of these genes may lead to abnormal differentiation, one consequence of which may be leukemia [16,18,38]. Table 1 summarizes the properties of these two major classes of type-C viruses;

TABLE 1. Distinguishing Features between Class I and Class II Type-C RNA Tumor Viruses

	Class I	Class II
Source	Usually normal tissues; can be neoplastic tissues.	Usually neoplastic tissues.
Oncogenicity	Generally not known to be oncogenic.	Generally known to be oncogenic.
Transmission	Usually vertical (germ line) as "provirus"; usually not infectious.	Usually horizontal but can infect germ line and be vertically transmitted.
Molecular Hybridization	RNA genome complexes to DNA from uninfected cell.	RNA genome complexes poorly to DNA from uninfected cell.

Table 2 lists the primate viruses we have grouped into the two classes; and Figure 1 schematically depicts the origin and genetic modification of type-C viruses.

In some species the class 1 and class 2 viruses are closely related. (By related 3 criteria have been particularly used, antigenic relatedness of reverse transriptase, antigenic relatedness of the p30 protein, and nucleotide sequence relatedness of the RNA genome.) Examples incude the avian viruses where RAV_0 (class 1) is related to AMV and RSV (class 2) and the murine viruses where the endogenous murine viruses (class 1) are related to the mouse leukemia and sarcoma viruses (class 2). In these cases we think the class 2 viruses evolved from the class 1. In contrast, in felines and primates the class 1 and 2 viruses are not related; presumably they have independent origins. These topics are discussed in detail in the paper by Dr. Todaro.

Primate Type-C RNA Tumor Viruses

Primates illustrate the two classes of type-C RNA tumor viruses described above. The class 1 example is an endogenous type-C virus originally isolated from baboon placenta and later induced from various normal tissues [59]. It has not been shown to be oncogenic. It is not surprising then that molecules related to endogenous molecules contained in this virus have been found in neoplastic *and normal* human tissues [52,59] as well as in other subhuman primates [38,59]. It will also not be surprising if the whole virus (endogenous) is induced from human cells. An alternative interpretation is that these proteins are not from an endogenous human type-C virus related to the endogenous baboon virus but are derived from infection of human cells with the baboon virus itself. In any case, these observations should not be overinterpreted as indicating that the virus or virus components are causatively involved in neoplasia. This remains to be proven for class 1 viruses.

In contrast, type-C viruses which are typical class 2 viruses have also been isolated from primates [33,56]. These viruses or components of these viruses have been usually detected in *neoplastic tissues* of primates. One was isolated from a fibrosarcoma of a woolly monkey or simian sarcoma virus (SSV). When injected into some recipient primates, it has induced sarcomas [10]. Others were isolated from gibbon apes. Gibbon ape leukemia virus (GaLV) was isolated both from lymphomas, lymphoid leukemias, and from myelogenous leukemia. Injection of the virus from gibbon myelogenous leukemia into newborn gibbons can sometimes induce myelogenous leu-

TABLE 2. Primate Type-C Oncornaviruses (RNA Tumor Viruses)

Virus	How Isolated	Class	Components Found in Normal Tissues	Proven Oncogenic
Baboon	Normal placenta cocultivated with heterologous cells Also induced from normal testes, lung, and kidney	1	Yes	No
Gibbon (GALV)	Several isolates. Some from a lymphoma, others from myelogenous or lymphoid leukemia. Some from normal brain.*	2	Not usual	Yes
Woolly (SSV)	Fibrosarcoma	2	Not usual	Yes

* Isolates from "normal" brains came from gibbons inoculated with extracts of human brain from patients with Kuru. See G. Todaro, elsewhere in this seminar.

kemia [30]. Despite the divergent evolutionary history of the species from which the woolly monkey virus (a new world primate) and the gibbon ape virus (an old world primate) were isolated, these two viruses are remarkably closely related by three tests (p30 protein; reverse transcriptase immunological cross reactivity; and nucleotide sequences of their RNA genome). There is evidence that these viruses originated in the distant past from a murine virus. This is supported by the recent isolate of a type-C (probably class 1) virus from an Asian mouse by Lieber et al. [36] which is closely related to SSV and GaLV (see Todaro's chapter in this seminar), and by our finding of an unusual relatedness of the RNA genome of SSV to DNA of normal uninfected mice [62]. In any event, these viruses are now infectious agents for at least 2 species of primates. Moreover, there may be an interesting relationship to man since (1) the primates from which virus was isolated were all in close contact with man and many were even injected with human material, and (2) proteins related to these viruses have been found in human tissues (see below). Table 2 summarizes some of the properties and history of these primate oncornaviruses.

Type-C Virus Components in Fresh Human Leukemia Blood Cells

Some electron microscopic observations in the past indicated that a small number of virus particles might be present in some human leukemia cells, but the observations were always controversial and the virus never isolated. For this reason in 1970 we began a systematic study of human leukemic cells to see if we could detect components of these viruses. We used molecular probes which would be advantageous for two reasons: greater sensitivity than microscopy, and if fully formed virus particles were not present we might find virion components or "footprints" of the virus. We and others have for the most part used four approaches: (1) determining if structures with biophysical properties (size, density, core structures, etc.) of oncornaviruses were present in the cell, i.e., as defective particles not released; (2) identification of reverse transcriptase, the virion specific DNA polymerase; (3) identification of viral RNA (by its size which is larger than cytoplasmic cellular RNA and its nucleotide sequence relatedness to RNA of human animal oncornaviruses); and (4) identification of the group specific (gs) antigen (p30 protein), a viral specific internal protein. Viral RNA and p30 protein are often found without an assembled virus, but generally reverse transcriptase is found only when virions are assembled, although this is not certain.

A. *Reverse Transcriptase*. After the discovery of reverse transcriptase in RNA tumor viruses [3,55], we reported detection of a similar activity in human leukemic cells [23]. This was the first description of this enzyme in any cell. However, we could not at that time conclude that this was viral reverse transcriptase since there was insufficient knowledge about the properties of this DNA polymerase in viruses and insufficient information about the properties of the three or more DNA polymerases of normal uninfected mammalian cells. Moreover, the identification of reverse transcriptase in cells is immeasurably more difficult than in viruses because of its very low activity, and much greater initial contamination with other proteins (most troublesome is the contamination with proteases and nucleases, which can distort polymerase activities, and also with other cellular polymerases and confuse the assays). Sensitivity and relative purity were required. Therefore, between 1970 and 1972 we purified reverse transcriptase from various RNA tumor viruses to get a detailed picture of their properties [1,17,22,44], and we isolated, partially purified, and characterized the DNA polymerases of normal human leukocytes [22,34,35,51]. We also obtained more detailed information about the properties of the enzyme in human leukemic cells [21,47,60]. These studies enabled us to conclude that: (1) the enzyme when identified and purified from human leukemia cells has the known biochemical and biophysical properties of reverse transcriptase from mammalian RNA tumor viruses [46]; (2) the enzyme was found in only 20–30% of patients with leukemia; (3) the enzyme could not be detected in normal fresh blood leukocytes, normal PHA stimulated lymphocytes, or normal human lymphoblast cell lines; (4) the enzyme in human leukemic cells was located in the cytoplasm in a particle which exhibited biophysical properties similar to those of an assembled RNA tumor virus [15,19,20]; and (5) within the particle the enzyme (prior to its purification away from the particle and other cellular elements) catalyzed an endogenous synthesis of DNA from an RNA template [15,19,20].

The questions, of course, then became to which animal virus was this protein related and what was the nature of the RNA template? These questions were answered between 1973 and 1974 with the availability of the primate viruses in sufficient quantity. George Todaro and I found that among all the RNA tumor viruses examined, the reverse transcriptase of human myelogenous leukemia cells was strongly related to reverse transcriptase from the gibbon ape leukemia virus and the woolly monkey sarcoma virus [60]. Reverse transcriptase was purified from various RNA tumor viruses (avian, murine, feline, and primate with representatives from both class 1 and class 2 viruses) and injected into rabbits and rats. Antibodies (IgG) were purified from the sera of these animals and used in assays designed to determine the amount of antibody required to neutralize the reverse transcriptase activity. Only antibodies to reverse transcriptase from the gibbon and woolly viruses strongly neutralized the enzyme from human myelogenous leukemia cells, and the inhibition curves indicated that the antigenic relatedness were very close. Less cross reaction was found with the antibody to reverse transcriptase from murine leukemia virus and little or none with other antibodies. This was then extended to several additional patients with acute myelogenous leukemia [15,19]. We should emphasize that this has been so far only demonstrated in adult acute myelogenous leukemia (AML). In other leukemias when we were successful in biochemically identifying this enzyme, we were unable to show antigenic relatedness to reverse transcriptase from any virus.

Because there has been confusion in the literature about reverse transcriptase in cells, I have summarized the criteria we use in Table 3, and especially since it is often confused with DNA polymerase γ, I have summarized the properties of this and the other polymerases of normal cells in Table 4, and compared their properties to reverse transcriptase.

B. *Viral-Related Nucleic Acid.* With the reverse transcriptase partially

TABLE 3. Criteria for Reverse Transcriptase

Biochemical Criteria
1. The enzyme activity is detected in particle fraction with a density of 1.16 gm/ml and shifted to 1.25 gm/ml upon treatment of adequate concentration of nonionic detergent.
2. The endogenous reaction requires all four deoxyribonucleotide triphosphates sensitive to RNase at least partically and resistant to actinomycin D, and product analysis reveals that the DNA is hydrogen bonded to a large RNA and covalently attached to a small RNA.
3. The purified enzyme is able to use oligo(dG)·(rC) and oligo(dT)·(rA) as template-primer but not oligo(dT)·(dA). When unpurified enzyme is used, the oligo(dT)·(rA) to oligo(dT)·(dA) ratio is high with Mg^{++} or Mn^{++} as divalent cation.
4. The enzyme is capable of transcribing heteropolymeric portions of 70S RNA.
5. The enzyme activity is stimulated by nonionic detergent when $(dT)_{oligo}·(rA)_n$, $(dT)_m·(rA)_n$, activated DNA or $(dG)_{oligo}·(rC)$ is used as template-primer.
6. The size of the enzyme is for mammalian type-C viruses, 160,000 daltons for most avian type-C and 110,000 daltons for type-B virus or MPMV.

Immunologic Criteria
   The enzyme activity is inhibited by purified IgG made against some known viral reverse transcriptase and not significantly inhibited by IgG against cellular DNA polymerases.

purified and characterized, the cytoplasmic "particles" that contain reverse transcriptase were examined to study the associated RNA molecule. High molecular weight RNA with some sequences related to the RNA of mouse leukemia virus strain Rauscher (RLV) [but not to that from avian myeloblastosis virus (AMV) nor mouse mammary tumor virus (MMTV)] was discovered in leukemic cells by Spiegelman and his colleagues [7,29,56]. We confirmed these observations [20,40] and then designed experiments to test by molecular hybridization the relatedness of the DNA synthesized by the reverse transcriptase in the cytoplasm of myelogenous leukemia cells to several RNA tumor viruses. We were looking for an "affinity pattern," i.e., if the human viral-related cytoplasmic nucleic acid contained sequences which complexed to the RNA of various RNA tumor viruses in a manner resembling the order of one of the animal viruses. (These experiments are done by synthesizing radio-labeled DNA, via the endogenous reverse transcriptase reaction. This DNA will contain sequences complementary to its template, the RNA in the particle. This DNA is used to hybridize to RNA from different viruses, and it reflects at least a portion of the sequences in the RNA template.) We did find that the RNA in human myelogenous leukemia cells (associated with reverse transcriptase) when matched with other RNA tumor viruses follows a pattern qualitatively like woolly sarcoma virus [19,20,40]. The relatedness of both the reverse transcriptase and the RNA in the cytoplasmic particles from these human cells to the analogous components in primate oncogenic (class 2) RNA tumor viruses has been demonstrated so far only with human myelogenous leukemia. These findings have recently been confirmed by 2 other groups [37,53].

C. *P30 Protein*. Two additional significant findings with fresh peripheral blood leukemic leukocytes then followed. First, Baxt et al. reported that the DNA of human leukemic cells contain sequences not found in normal leukocytes [6], and these sequences are viral-related [5]. These findings imply an infectious process. Second, Sherr and Todaro recently found a protein in 5 cases of acute myelogenous leukemia [49] antigenically related to p30 protein of woolly sarcoma virus and gibbon ape leukemia virus. The relative relationships between the viral components in human leukemic cells and those from animal RNA tumor viruses are compared in summary form in Table 5.

In summary, three components were identified in peripheral blood human myelogenous leukemia cells specifically related to analogous components in oncogenic (class 2) primate type-C RNA tumor viruses. These findings combined with the evidence for extra (unique) sequences reported in human leukemic cells are most simply interpreted as arguing for the addition of

TABLE 4. Classification and Properties of Mammalian DNA Polymerases Obtained Specifically from Human Cells[a]

Human leukemic	DNA polymerase α	DNA polymerase β	DNA polymerase γ	reverse transcriptase
Cellular location (suspected)	Cytoplasm	Nucleus or cytoplasm	Unknown	Cytoplasm
Molecular weight	1.3×10^5	0.4×10^5	$\sim 10^5$	1.3×10^5; 0.7×10^5[b]
Template-primer preference (under optimum conditions)	"Activated DNA" (Mg^{2+}); $dA_n \cdot dT\overline{15} \gg rA_n \cdot dT\overline{15}$ (Mn^{2+} or Mg^{2+})	$dA_n \cdot dT\overline{15} \geq rA_n \cdot dT\overline{15}$ (Mn^{2+}); $dA_n \cdot dT\overline{15} > rA_n \cdot dT15$ (MG^{2+})	$dA_n \cdot dT\overline{15} < rA_n \cdot dT\overline{15}$ (Mn^{2+})[c]; $dA_n \cdot dT\overline{15} > rA_n \cdot dT15$ (Mg^{2+})[c]	$dA_n \cdot dT\overline{15} \ll rA_n \cdot dT\overline{15}(MN^{2+})$[d]
Utilization of heteropolymeric regions of HMW viral RNA	None	None	Slight or none	Moderate or strong
Inhibition with antibody (IgG) prepared against purified DNA polymerases from:				
SiSV or GaLV	None	None	None	Strong
MuLV[k]	None	None	None	Weak
FeLV, AvLV, or MpMV[k]	None	None	None	None
DNA polymerase-α cells	Strong	None	None	None
Previous names; see footnote:				
[e]	DNA polymerase I	DNA polymerase II	DNA polymerase III	
[f]	DNA polymerase II	DNA polymerase I	R DNA polymerase	
[g]	Maxi DNA polymerase	Mini DNA polymerase		
[h]	Cytoplasmic DNA polymerase	N_1 DNA polymerase		
[i]	DNA polymerase C	DNA polymerase N	A DNA polymerase	
[j]	6-8 S DNA polymerase	3.5 S DNA polymerase		

(a) Nomenclature of vertebrate DNA polymerases according to the conventions developed by D. Baltimore, F. J. Bollum, R. C. Gallo, and A. Weissbach at a meeting on May 29, 1974, and proposed for general use. It was agreed that there is sufficient evidence of distinct molecular properties and template specificities to name five different types of DNA polymerases associated with vertebrate, in particular mammalian, tissues. The three cellular RNA polymerases are named α, β, γ in the chronological order of discovery in order to minimize controversy and confusion arising from overlapping properties and from conflicting uses of I, II, and III. The viral DNA polymerase ("reverse transcriptase") was considered to be a special case and no specific recommendation was made. The mitochondrial DNA polymerase, distinctly associated with mitochondria, is called simple "mitochondrial DNA polymerase"; there are also distinguishing properties for this enzyme (see footnote f). (Note: dT15 is used in place of the usual dT12-18.)

(b) The 1.3×10^5 form is converted to a 0.7×10^5 form in high salt (H. Mondal, R. E. Gallagher and R. C. Gallo, unpublished observations).

(c) $dA_n \cdot dT15$ activity with Mg^{2+} is occasionally comparable to that of $rA_n \cdot dT15$ with Mn^{2+}.

(d) Occasional preparations have equally high activity with $(rC)_n \cdot (dG)15$.

(e) R. G. Smith and R. C. Gallo, 1972, PNAS 69: 2879; B. J. Lewis, J. Abrell, R. Smith and R. Gallo, 1974, Science 183: 867–869.

(f) M. Fry and A. Weissbach, 1973, Biochem. 12: 3602–3608.

(g) M. S. Coleman, J. J. Hutton and F. J. Bollum, 1974, Blood 44: 19.

(h) W. D. Sedwick, T. S.-F. Wang and D. Korn, 1972, JBC 247: 5026.

(i) R. McCaffrey, D. F. Smoler and D. Baltimore, 1973, PNAS 70: 521.

(j) L. M. S. Chang and F. J. Bollum, 1972, JBC 247: 7948.

(k) MuLV is murine leukemia virus. FeLV is feline leukemia virus. AvLV is avian leujemia virus. MpMV is Mason-Pfizer moneky virus, an oncornavirus more type-B than C, isolated from a rhesus breast carcinoma.

TABLE 5. Relative Relationships between Viral-like Components in Human Myelogenous Leukemic Cells and Analogous Components from Various Animal RNA Tumor Viruses

Human Virus-like Components

Reverse Transcriptase	Protein Related to p30 Protein	RNA Template for Reverse Transcriptase	Virus
+++	+++	not tested	Gibbon ape leukemia
−	+	−	Baboon endogenous
+	−	++	Mouse sarcoma-leukemia complex
+			
−	−	−	Cat endogenous (RD114)
−	−	−	Cat sarcoma
−	−	−	Cat leukemia
−	−	−	Avian sarcoma or leukemia

See references 15, 20, 41, and 60 for the detailed data on the immunologic relatedness of reverse transcriptase from myelogenous human leukemic cells to reverse transcriptases of animal viruses. The references for the relatedness of the RNA template to the animal virus RNA genome are 15, 19, 37, 40, and 53. The identification of the p30 protein in fresh human myelogenous leukemic cells and its specific relatedness to the p30 of woolly monkey sarcoma virus and gibbon ape leukemia virus were made by C. Sherr and G. Todaro [49].

information from these or a related virus, although more complex interpretations are possible. The epidemiology clearly indicates, however, that neither this nor any other cancer is contagious in the usual sense. Therefore, if indeed it is an infectious disease, it must involve a complicated mechanism, environmental factors in addition to virus, a very marked variation in host response, or a combination of these.

Continuous Growth and Differentiation of Human Myelogenous Leukemia Cells and Isolation of Type-C Virus

Recently, we identified a factor from one particular whole human embryo cell line which when added to human myelogenous leukemia cells (obtained from blood or bone marrow) promotes their exponential growth and differentiation in liquid suspension tissue culture [14]. The factor appears to be specific for these cells. For instance, normal myelogenous cells from bone marrow and lymphoid leukemia cells do not respond. The presence of the factor appears to be continuously required. From one patient (A.S.) budding type-C virus was identified after early passage of the cells [14,13,54]. The virus has now been identified in 4 separate cultures from 2 separate samples (blood and bone marrow) from this one patient [14]. As in several other patients with acute myelogenous leukemia, we had previously identified reverse transcriptase in the fresh blood myeloblasts from this patient. In fact, because of some biochemical studies which were in progress, the reverse transcriptase of this patient's blood myeloblasts was the subject of an earlier and separate report [41] prior to the virus isolation. As with previous studies with AML, the reverse transcriptase was immunologically very closely related to this enzyme from SSV and GaLV. Similarly, the reverse transcriptase [13,54] and p30 protein [54,50] of the isolated virus was also closely related to SSV and GaLV. In collaboration with N. Teich and R. Weiss of the Imperial Cancer Research Foundation in London, we have found that this virus infects cells of several species including man [54]. Figure 2 summarizes our virus isolates from this patient. Recently Nooter et al. identified a similar virus in a child with lymphosarcoma leukemia [42] and Gabelman et al. a similar virus in a patient with chronic lymphocytic leukemia [12]. A most striking observation was recently made by Panem et al. [43]. They report several isolates of type-C virus from several normal human embryos. If these findings can be verified they will be a landmark discovery, implying to me that the source of virus is by congenital infection. This would be consistent with the lack of epidemiologic evidence for infection. Finally, there is one interesting clinical observation which is most consistent with a transmissable agent being causatively involved in the disease. Don Thomas and his colleagues in Seattle have been ablating the bone marrow of leukemic patients and then attempting to graft them with normal donor bone marrow. In 2 of 6 original cases, apparently the normal donor cells underwent leukemic transformation after inoculation into the recipient leukemia patient [57]. A third instance has been recently found [58]. One major problem with the virus isolates is that so far we have not been able is to identify the complete provirus in human leukemic cells. Although there are several possible reasons for this, the data cannot be contrued as strong evidence that these viruses are causatively involved in this disease until this is achieved.

Pathogenesis (Phenotypic Change)

Most workers believe that in AML the physiologic abnormality is with the process of differentiation of the granulocyte precursors, e.g., myelo-

TISSUE CULTURE PASSAGES AND MEDIA DNA POLYMERASE ASSAYS FROM HUMAN ACUTE MYELOGENOUS LEUKEMIA CELLS (PATIENT HL–23)

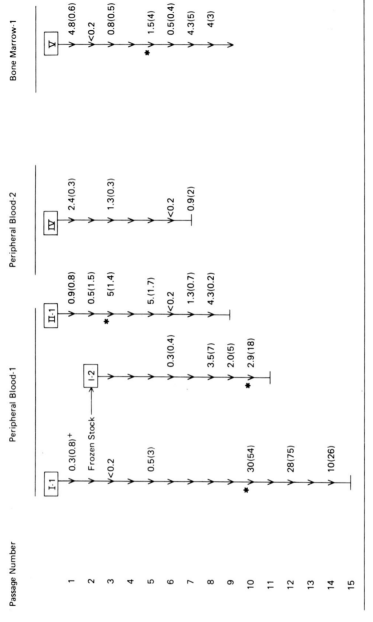

* Passage at which type-C virus was identified by EM.

† Numbers indicate pmoles TMP incorporated/ml tissue culture fluid/hr. Numbers in parentheses indicate the ratio of polymerase activity with oligo(dT)-poly(A) to oligo-(dT)-poly(dA).

blasts, to the mature polymorphonuclear leukocytes or between stem cells and committed granulocyte precursor cells. This is often viewed as a "block" in differentiation, and it has been discussed in detail previously by many workers. Studies from many laboratories have shown that there are substances released into the medium from some cells which when added to hemopoietic cells can induce modest temporary growth and differentiation of these cells, especially on a solid matrix. "Factors" which have this effect have been called colony stimulating activity (CSA) and MGI (macrophage granulocyte inducer), and the systems were first developed by Sachs and his colleagues (see reference 58 for a review) and by Metcalf, Moore and their coworkers [39]. Using these materials, some studies have indicated that the phenotypic abnormality in AML is reversible, i.e., they respond to the putative regulator molecules and differentiate. Others believe that the arrest in differentiation is irreversible. The picture which appears to be emerging is that the population of AML cells is heterogenous in this respect, some respond and others cannot [2]. Does this mean that the genetic change (if any) which leads to leukemic transformation is present in only a fraction of the cells we call leukemic, or is it present in all cells but expressed (DNA RNA) to a varying degree in different leukemic cells? This is an unanswered but important question. In any case these and other studies have shown that, at minimum, a fraction of AML cells do apparently respond normally to these stimuli. In addition, the "factor" recently discovered in our laboratory (see above) which appears to be specific for myelogenous leukemia cells promotes continuous exponential growth of these cells and maturation of at least some of them in liquid suspension culture. It has no affect on ALL, CLL, or normal bone marrow or peripheral blood cells. This "factor" differs from the CSA described to date because: (1) of its specificity for leukemic cells while CSA works best or more predictably on normal cells; (2) of its induction of exponential growth; (3) its affect can be maintained continuously; (4) it works on cells in suspension and has no effect promoting colony formation on the agar plate system. The difference between the response of the leukemic and normal cells again emphasizes a cellular difference between the two. Since some of these results were obtained with

---

FIG. 2 (see facing page). Summary of the virus isolates from patient HL-23 (or A.S.) with acute myelogenous leukemia. Peripheral blood sample 1 was obtained in Oct. 1973, blood sample-2 in Dec. 1974, and bone marrow-1 in Feb. 1975. The numbers to the right of the arrows indicate the DNA polymerase activity in pmoles TMP incorporated/ml tissue culture fluid/hour, using oligo(dT)·poly(A) as primer-template. Details are described elsewhere [16]. The numbers in parentheses are the ratios of polymerase activity with oligo(dT)·poly(A) to oligo(dT)·poly(dA) of material pelleted from the media. In our hands, ratios above 2 of media samples are suggestive of detection of viral reverse transcriptase and significantly higher values are almost invariably due to viral reverse transcriptase [53].

leukemic cells containing marker chromosomes and since normal cells do not respond to this "factor," we believe these results substantially add to the evidence that at least some leukemic (AML) cells can be induced to differentiate.

What is the cellular change responsible for the above mentioned functional differenes between normal and leukemic cells? Despite many morphological, immunological, and biochemical studies, this has not been pinpointed in AML or in any other neoplasia. For theoretical reasons many workers suspect the membrane. It is also attractive to view the above mentioned differences in the response of normal and myelogenous leukemic cells to the growth and differentiation inducing factors as differences in membrane recognition of these factors. Direct support for a change in the surface of transformed cells comes from reports of differences in response to certain lectins of murine leukemic and other transformed cells compared to normal cells [45]. However, I am not aware of any substantial study of this with human leukemic cells. Probably, the best evidence that the surface of leukemic cells differs from normal are recent results of Billings et al. [8] and particularly of Greaves [26] on isolation of a leukemia specific surface antigen. Some exciting avenues of research for the future should include studies directed to substantiating these findings, determining if they contribute to the abnormality in differentiation, and determine if these membrane antigens are viral structural proteins or viral induced.

REFERENCES

1. Abrell JW, Gallo RC: J Virol 12: 431, 1973.
2. Aye MT, Till JE, McCulloch E: Blood 45: 485, 1975.
3. Baltimore D: Nature 226: 1209, 1970.
4. Battula N, Loeb LA: J Biol Chem 249: p. 4086, 1974.
5. Baxt W: Proc Natl Acad Sci USA 71: 2853, 1974.
6. Baxt W, Hehlman R, Spiegelman S: Nature [New Biol] 244: 72, 1972.
7. Baxt WG, Spiegelman S: Proc Natl Acad Sci USA 69: 3737, 1972.
8. Billings, R, Terasaki P: In Neth R (Ed): Modern Trends in Human Leukemia, II. (In press).
9. Dahlberg JE, Harada F, Sawyer RC: In DNA Synthesis in Vitro. Cold Spring Harbor Symp Quant Biol, Vol. 39, Part 2, 1974, p 925.
10. Deinhardt F: Personal communication.
11. Essex M: In Advances in Cancer Research, vol. 21. New York, Academic Press, 1975, p 175.
12. Gabelman N, Waxman S, Smith W, et al: Int J Cancer (in press).
13. Gallagher RE, Gallo RC: Science 187: 350, 1975.
14. Gallagher RE, Salahuddin SZ, Hall WT, et al: Proc Nat Acad Sci USA (in press).
15. Gallagher RE, Todaro GJ, Smith RG, et al: Proc Nat Acad Sci USA 71: 1309, 1974.
16. Gallo RC: In Neth R, Gallo RC, Spiegelman S, Stohlman F (Eds): Modern Trends in Human Leukemia. Munich, J. F. Lehmanns Verlag, 1974, p. 227.

17. Gallo RC, Abrell JW, Robert MS, et al: J Natl Cancer Inst 49: 7, 1972.
18. Gallo RC, Gallagher RE: *In* Jensen KG, Killman SA, Gunz FW (Eds): Series Hae-matologica, The Etiology of Leukemia, volume 6. Copenhagen, Munksgaard, 1974, p 224.
19. Gallo RC, Gallagher RE, Miller NR, et al: *In* Cold Spring Harbor Symp Quant Biol: Tumor Viruses, Vol. 39, 1975, p 933.
20. Gallo RC, Miller NR, Saxinger WC, Gillespie D: Proc Natl Acad Sci USA 70: 3219, 1973.
21. Gallo RC, Sarin PS, Sarngadharan MG, et al: *In* Beers RF (Ed): Proc Sixth Miles International Symposium on Molecular Biology. Baltimore, Johns Hopkins University Press, 1973, p 180.
22. Gallo RC, Sarin PS, Smith RG, et al: *In* Wess R, Inman R (Eds): DNA Synthesis *in Vitro.* Proc 2nd Annual Steenbock Symposium. Baltimore, University Park Press, 1973, p 251.
23. Gallo RC, Yang SS, Ting RC: Nature 228: p. 927, 1970.
24. Gillespie D, Gallo RC: Science 188: 802, 1975.
25. Gillespie D, Saxinger WC, Gallo RC: *In* Progress in Nucleic Acid Research and Molecular Biology, Vol. 15. New York Academic Press, 1975, p 1.
26. Greaves M: *In* Neth R (Ed.): Modern Trends in Human Leukemia, II (in press).
27. Green M, Gerard G: *In* Cohn WE (Ed): Progress and Nucleic Acid Research and Molecular Biology, Vol. 14, 1974, p 187.
28. Gross L: *In* Oncogenic Viruses (ed 2). London, Pergamon Press, 1970.
29. Hehlmann R, Kufe D, Spiegelman S: Proc Natl Acad Sci USA 69: 435, 1972.
30. Kawakami TG, Buckley PM, Coggan RJ, et al: Proc Am Soc Clin Path p. 110, 1974.
31. Kawakami TG, Huff SD, Buckley PM, et al: Nature [New Biol] 235: 170, 1972.
32. Lerner R: Personal communication.
33. Levy JA: Science 182: 1151, 1973.
34. Lewis BJ, Abrell JW, Smith RG, Gallo RC: Science 183: 867, 1974.
35. Lewis BJ, Abrell JW, Smith RG, Gallo RC: Biochim Biophys Acta 349: 148, 1974.
36. Lieber MM, Sherr CJ, Todaro GJ, et al: Proc Natl Acad Sci USA (in press).
37. Mak TW, Kurtz S, Manaster J, et al: Proc Natl Acad Sci USA 72: 623, 1975.
38. Mayer RJ, Smith RG, Gallo RC: Science 185: 764, 1974.
39. Metcalf D, Bradley TR, Robinson W: J Cell Physiol 69: 93, 1967.
40. Miller NR, Saxinger WC, Reitz MS, et al: Proc Natl Acad Sci USA 71: 3177, 1974.
41. Mondal H, Gallagher RE, Gallo RC: Proc Natl Acad Sci USA 72: 1194, 1975.
42. Nooter K, Aarsen AM, Bentvelzen P, et al: Nature (in press).
43. Panem S, Prochownik E, Reale F, Kirsten W: Science (in press).
44. Robert MS, Smith RG, Gallo RC, et al: Science 176: 798, 1972.
45. Sachs L: Harvey Lectures, Series 68. New York, Academic Press 1974, p 1.
46. Sarin PS, Gallo RC: *In* Burton K (Ed): International Review of Science, Chapter 8, Vol. 6. Oxford, Butterworth and Medical and Technical Publishing Co., 1974, p 219.
47. Sarngadharan MG, Sarin PS, Reitz MS, Gallo RC: Nature [New Biol] 240: 67, 1972.
48. Scolnick EM, Maryak JM, Parks WP: J Virol 14: 1435, 1974.
49. Sherr C, Todaro GJ: Science 187: 855, 1975.
50. Sherr C, Todaro G; and Aaronson S, Gilden R: Unpublished data.
51. Smith RG, Gallo RC: Proc Natl Acad Sci USA 69: 2879, 1972.
52. Strand M, August JT: J Virol 14: 1584, 1974.
53. Tavitian A: Personal communication.
54. Teich NM, Weiss RA, Salahuddin SZ, et al: Nature (in press).
55. Temin HM, Mizutani S: Nature 226: 1211, 1970.
56. Theilen GH, Gould D, Fowler M, et al: J Natl Cancer Inst 47: 881, 1971.

57. Thomas ED, Storb RR, Clift RA, et al.: N Engl J Med 292: 832 and 805, 1975.
58. Thomas ED: Personal communication.
59. Todaro GJ, Benveniste RE, Callahan R, et al: *In* Cold Spring Harbor Symp Quant Biol: Tumor Viruses, Vol. 39, 1975, p 1159.
60. Todaro GJ, Gallo RC: Nature 244: 206, 1973.
61. Weiss RA: *In* Nakahara W, Hirayama T, Nishioka K, Sugano H (Eds): Analytical and Experimental Epidemiology of Cancer. Baltimore, University Park Press, 1973, p 201.
62. Wong-Staal F, Gallo RC, Gillespie D: Nature (in press).

The Relationship of Chromosomal Abnormalities to Neoplasia

Janet D. Rowley, M.D.

One of the major questions that remains to be answered in neoplasia is the relationship of the observed chromosomal changes to the initiation and evolution of the malignant state. A consistent chromosome abnormality has been observed in bone marrow cells obtained from about 90% of patients with chronic myelogenous leukemia (CML).

On the other hand, a much lower percentage of patients with acute leukemia (AL) show marrow chromosomal abnormalities, and the pattern of changes is quite variable. This same variable problem has been observed in other human tumors. Therefore, the assumption has been made that the consistent change in CML is exceptional and that chromosomal abnormalities in AL and most human tumors are merely epiphenomena.

These observations are derived from studies in which conventional staining procedures have been used that do not permit identification of individual chromosomes. The new staining techniques using quinacrine fluorescence [1] and Giemsa banding [19] that allow the precise identification of each human chromosome have been used to reexamine the question of the variability of chromosomal changes in human tumors.

Most of the data relevant to this question have been obtained from studies of patients with hematologic abnormalities, particularly acute and chronic myelogenous leukemia.

The analyses are done on bone marrow cells, within an hour of the time of aspiration, which avoids the problem of cell selection in culture. The cells are examined with quinacrine fluorescense, and the precise abnormality is determined by this procedure. The analysis is very time consuming, particularly when one studies leukemic cells in which the pattern of bands may be indistinct.

The study of chromosomes in human tumors received its first boost from the observation in 1960 by Nowell and Hungerford [11] that marrow cells from patients with CML contained a consistent abnormality. One of the small chromosomes appeared to have a deletion of about two-thirds of its

From The University of Chicago, Division of the Biological Sciences, and the Pritzker School of Medicine, Chicago, Ill.

long arm; this marker chromosome was called the Philadelphia or Ph[1] chromosome. Whether the material was lost from the cell, or whether it was translocated to another chromosome, could not be determined at that time due to our inability to identify each chromosome precisely. The Ph[1] chromosome is found in about 90% of patients with CML [20]. Cultured lymphocytes from these patients show a normal karyotype (chromosomal pattern). Therefore, the abnormality resulting in the Ph[1] chromosome represents a somatic mutation in an otherwise chromosomally normal individual.

In 1970, quinacrine fluorescence analysis showed that the Ph[1] was a chromosome 22 [2,13]. As I examined cells from patients with CML, I observed that, in fact, there was a second consistent abnormality in these patients. In addition to the small number 22, every one of the 45 patients that I have analyzed has had an additional band of material at the end of chromosome No. 9 [14]. This abnormal No. 9 is referred to as the 9 q+ chromosome ("q" refers to the long arm of a chromosome). The pattern of the fluorescent bands, and the amount of additional material, suggested that this was the piece missing from the Ph[1] chromosome. Recently, I have collaborated with Dr. Mortimer Mendelsohn and his group at Livermore Laboratories. He developed the use of a DNA-specific stain to measure the DNA content of individual chromosomes [9]. In this project, I analyze the cells with quinacrine fluorescence, and the group at Livermore stained the same cells and determined the DNA content of each chromosome. This technic has shown that the Ph[1] chromosome has lost 0.40 units of DNA (or 45%) when compared with the normal No. 22, whereas the 9q+ chromosome contains 0.42 units more DNA than a normal No. 9 [7]. This indicates that no chromosomal material has been lost, and provides further confirmation of the presumptive translocation.

In addition to the 45 patients with CML whom I have analyzed, I know of about 150 more who have been studied. All of my patients, as well as the great majority of the others, have the translocation to the end of No. 9. There are a few exceptions; I know of eight at the present time [3,4,5,10,12]. The exceptional translocations have involved the end of the long arm of No. 2, the short arm of No. 3, the long arm of No. 5, the long arm of No. 10, the long arm of No. 17, a No. 19, and an unidentified chromosome. Present evidence indicates that about 95% of all patients have the specific 9q+, 22q-translocation.

This is the only example of such a specific translocation that has been observed in humans. The mechanism for producing such a specific translocation is obscure. It may be that these chromosomes are located adjacent to each other in the cell and that this proximity predisposes to the translocation. It is also possible that these chromosomes contain homologous sequences of DNA, which increase the frequency of rearrangements. Each of these suggestions should lead to an increased frequency of this translocation in all cells, which would be observed as a constitutional chromosomal abnormality; but such is not the case! I suspect the explanation must be looked for elsewhere. A further dilemma is finding an explanation for the malignant behavior of these CML cells. Originally, when it was assumed that the Ph[1] was a deletion, one could propose that the loss of certain genes regulating the proliferation of myeloid cells resulted in the neoplastic change. Since it has been shown that there is no such loss, another explanation must be sought. One possibility is that, although Ph[1] positive cells contain the normal amount of DNA, this DNA becomes functionally inactive as a result of the translocation. This would be the first example of a position effect in man, if this is the correct explanation.

Whereas the chromosomal pattern in CML has appeared to be quite consistent, with approximately 90% of patients having the Ph[1] chromosome, such consistency has not been observed in acute leukemia. Chromosomal abnormalities have been detected in about 40% of the patients; the number of chromosomes has ranged from 23 to over 100, and the pattern has appeared to be quite variable. It is no wonder that investigators assumed that the chromosomal changes were an epiphenomenon. Newer evidence obtained from studies of banded chromosomes suggest that this view is wrong. Twenty-five of 50 patients with acute leukemia studied in my laboratory have an abnormal karyotype. Careful fluorescence analysis of cells from these patients has shown several groups with similar abnormalities. In three of these, the chromosome number was 45. The original Giemsa analysis suggested that these patients were lacking two C group chromosomes and a G, and had an extra D and an extra E instead. Quinacrine fluorescence revealed that these patients who were females were lacking an X. In addition, each patient had a break in one chromosome, No. 8, in the same band (8q22). In two of the patients, the end of No. 8 was translocated to the end of the long arm of No. 21 [15]; in the third, it was translocated to the end of the long arm of No. 17 [16]. Whereas these data provided some evidence for nonrandom abnormalities, a recent paper [18] reported two more patients with the same 8/21 translocation just described. This report also mentioned 9 other patients whose karyotypic pattern was compatible with an 8/21 translocation, although the cells have not been examined with any banding technics. I think this provides one piece of evidence that chromosome abnormalities in acute leukemia are nonrandom.

The best evidence for nonrandom involvement of chromosomes, not only in leukemia, but in other hematologic disorders as well, comes from an analysis of the extra C group chromosomes (X and pairs 6 through 12) so frequently found in these diseases. When patients with CML enter the acute

TABLE 1. Author's data: number of patients showing C group abnormalities

Disorder	\-7	\-X	+X	+8	+9	+10	+11
			Chromosome abnormality				
CML-acute phase			(1)*	6		(1)*	
AL	1	3		5			1
PV	1†			1	1(1)*		
Other	1			1			
Total	3	3	(1)	13	1(1)	(1)	1

* ( ) In addition to no. 8.
† Lacks 7q distal to 7q22 (q = long arm of a chromosome).
(Proc. Natl. Acad. Sci. USA 72: 152, 1975.)

Table 2. All data: number of patients showing C group abnormalities

Disorder	\-7	\-9	\-X	+X	+7	+8	+9	+10	+11	+12
				Chromosome abnormality						
CML-acute				(1)*	(1)†	7		1(1)*		1
Ph¹ negative								1		
AL	4	1	4(1)*			10	1		2	
PV	1‡					4	2(3)*			
Other	2§					6	3			
Total	7¶	1	4(1)	(1)	(1)	28¶	6(3)¶	1(1)	2	1

* ( ) In addition to no. 8.
† ( ) In addition to no. 12.
‡ Lacks 7q distal to q22.
§ 7p distal to 7p11 is lacking in one patient (p = short arm of a chromosome).
¶ Chromosome is involved in loss or gain more frequently than would be expected ($P \leqq 0.008$).
Refs.: personal communication from (a) Van den Berghe, H.; (b) de la Chapelle, A.; (c) Pan, S. F.; and (d) Lin, C. C.
Proc. Natl. Acad. Sci. USA 72: 152, 1975.)

phase, one of the most common changes is the addition of one or more C group chromosomes. I have examined 6 such patients; each had the same extra chromosome, namely No. 8. Three patients had two extra C's, the second one being an 8, a 10, or an X (in a male). Thus it is possible, at last, to distinguish random from nonrandom changes. Of the six patients with AML who had additional C's, cells from five could be analyzed with fluorescence and every patient showed an extra No. 8. I have examined cells from three patients with hematologic problems other than leukemia, and have identified one with an extra No. 8, one with an extra No. 8 and No. 9 and one with a No. 9 [17] (See Table 1). Thus an extra No. 8 is the most common abnormality regardless of the clinical disorder. My data, plus those published from other laboratories, are summarized in Table 2 and Figure 1. The numbers are greater, but the interpretation is the same.

I should point out that this nonrandomness is not restricted to diseases of the bone marrow. It has been known for some time that cells in most meningiomas are lacking a chromosome No. 22 [6]. When these cells lose chro-

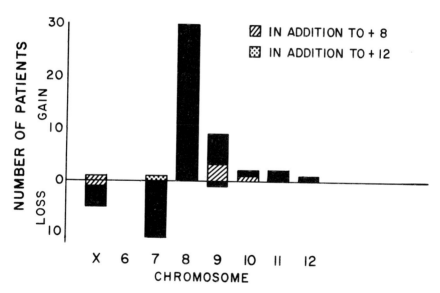

FIG. 1. The data from the 21 patients recorded in Table 1, plus the 29 patients with a variety of hematologic disorders studied by other laboratories (Table 2) are summarized in this figure. The black portion of a column represents patients who have gained or lost chromosomes, shown above or below the line, respectively. The hatched area represents patients who have a second C group abnormality, in addition to an extra No. 8, and the dotted area is the single patient who had an extra No. 7 as well as a No. 12. It is clear that when patients gain chromosomes, they are most often No. 8, and less often a No. 9; when chromosomes are lost, a No. 7, and less frequently an X in females, are involved.

mosomes (which they do much more often than gaining them), the one most frequently lost is No. 8; No. 1 is next, and then No. 9. Patients with diseases of the lymphatic system, such as Burkitt's lymphoma, multiple myeloma, and ataxia telangiectasia, show abnormalities of chromosome 14 [8]. Polyps of the colon have an extra 14 and, in one patient, an extra No. 8 as well. On the basis of present data, it appears that only some chromosomes are abnormal, and that these chromosomes are affected in a variety of tumors or somatic mutations.

One is faced with the question of the meaning of these observations. Analysis of the work done on the production of tumors in experimental animals can provide a model which may apply to the nonrandom chromosomal abnormalities that I have described.

Two important conclusions can be drawn from the animal work. First, both Rous Sarcoma Virus (RSV) and dimethylbenzanthracene (DMBA) produce sarcomas in the same strain of inbred rats; these tumors are histologically indistinguishable. The cytogeneticist, however, can tell them apart because the majority of tumors produced by RSV have one specific karyotype observed in the majority of tumors that is distinctly different than the specific karyotype produced by DMBA. Secondly, DMBA, if administered to the same species of rats by a different route, produces leukemia. The chromosomal pattern seen in these leukemic cells is virtually identical to that observed in the sarcomas. Thus the karyotypic change is agent-specific and is independent of the type of tumor produced.

The situation in man is admittedly much more complex. One major difference is the genetic heterogeneity in man compared with inbred strains of animals. Nevertheless, a similar model can be proposed for man [17]. We have identified specific karyotypic patterns, such as extra No. 8's or No. 9's. The same karyotypic change has been observed in histologically different disorders, represented here by leukemia, polycythemia vera, and anemias. The etiologic agents in these disorders are undetermined at present. It is possible that, when we have developed the appropriate technics for detecting the etiology agents in these diseases, we may find that one agent is associated with one specific karyotype, such as +8, and that another agent will be associated with a different specific karyotype, even though both etiologic agents could produce the same spectrum of clinical diseases. This model may be applicable to CML. In this situation, the Ph[1] positive form would have one etiology, whereas the Ph[1] negative variant would have a different etiology.

In conclusion, I have presented evidence that the Ph[1] chromosome represents a specific translocation rather than a deletion. Furthermore, there is evidence, even though preliminary, that other chromosome changes are nonrandom.

The frequent association of abnormalities of chromosome No. 8, as an extra chromosome or in a translocation, with hematologic disorders is perplexing. No. 8 is also abnormal in meningiomas and possibly in polyps of the colon. The significance of these observations is unclear.

Investigators can learn much from the relatively more controlled systems of carcinogenesis in inbred animals or *in vitro* tissue cultures, but I believe that a careful study of the chromosomal abnormalities found in our patients will provide important clues to the fundamental mechanisms of cancer in *man*.

REFERENCES

1. Caspersson T, Zech L, Johansson C, Modest EJ: Chromosoma 30: 215, 1970.
2. Caspersson TG, Lindsten J, et al: Exp Cell Res 63: 238, 1970.
3. Engel E, McGee BJ, Flexner JM, et al: N Engl J Med 291: 154, 1974.
4. Gahrton G, Zech L, Lindsten J: Exp Cell Res 86: 214, 1974.
5. Hayata I, Sakurai M, Kakati S, Sandbert A: Cancer 36: 1177–91, 1975.
6. Mark J, Levan G, Mitelman F: Hereditas 71: 163, 1972.
7. Mayall B, Carrano A, Rowley J: Clin Chem 20: 1080, 1974.
8. McCaw BK, Hecht F, Harnden DG, et al: Proc Natl Acad Sci USA 72: 2071, 1975.
9. Mendelsohn ML, Mayall BH, Bogart E, et al: Science 179: 1126, 1973.
10. Mitelman F: Hereditas 76: 315, 1974.
11. Nowell PC, Hungerford DA: Science 132: 1197, 1960.
12. Nowell PC, Jensen J, Gardner F: Humangenetik 30: 13–21, 1975.
13. O'Riordan, ML, Robinson JA, Buckton KE, et al: Nature 230: 167, 1971.
14. Rowley JD: Nature 243: 290, 1973.
15. Rowley JD: Ann Genet 16: 109, 1973.
16. Rowley JD: Lancet 2: 835, 1974.
17. Rowley JD: Proc Natl Acad Sci 72: 152, 1975.
18. Sakuri M, Oshimura M, Kahati S, Sandberg AA: Lancet 2: 227, 1974.
19. Sumner AT, Evans HJ, Buckland RA: Nature [New Biol] 232: 31, 1971.
20. Whang-Peng J, Canellos GP, Carbone PP, Tijo JH: Blood 32: 755, 1968.

Tumor-Specific Immunity

Richard T. Smith, M.D.

In this paper, current status of knowledge of immunologic relationships between growing tumor and host will be reviewed. The data from which these generalizations are derived involve studies of both autochtonous human tumors and animal systems in which the syngeneic relationship between tumor and host limits the antigenic differences to those specific to the tumor. Current information can be summarized in the oversimplified statement that most tumors present multiple antigenic and immunogenic determinants which are derived from the cell membranes. These antigens stimulate a polyclonal hyperimmune state in the host involving most or all elements of the immune response. It is a paradox that a primary tumor above a critical mass will continue to grow and will kill the host despite apparently competent specific immune mechanisms.

The presentation will deal with five elements of the tumor-host relationship: (1) the source and character of tumor antigens: (2) the fate and distribution of such antigens; (3) the components of the immune response which these tumor determinants evoke as determined by both *in vivo* and *in vitro* analysis; (4) the problems of blocking and application of *in vitro* analysis to the *in vivo* tumor-host relationship; and (5) a tentative synthesis suggesting a balanced relationship between growing tumor and host immune systems.

I. Tumor Antigens: Source and Quality

A long-standing dogma in tumor immunology holds that tumor antigens are of two types: (1) antigens (TSTA) associated with the tumor and having an apparent role in bringing about its specific rejection in an immune host; (2) antigens (TAA) which are tumor specific but appear not to provide targets for immunologic attack in appropriate *in vivo* systems. The test

From the Department of Pathology, University of Florida, Gainesville, Fla.

Supported in part by grants from RO NIH (HD-0083) (CA-04480) and a training grant from one NCI. The work described from our laboratory represents the collaborative efforts of J. Forbes, R. Blackstock, P. Klein, and R. Nowinski.

system which demonstrates the former (TSTA) involves the inoculation of small numbers of living tumor cells into a syngeneic host, amputating or otherwise removing the tumor after appropriate growth, then testing the recovered host for resistance to the original as compared to other tumors derived from that line. In such a test system, chemical carcinogen-induced tumors show a high degree of specificity in that only the homologous tumors—ones which induced the resistant state—will be rejected upon re-inoculation. Other syngeneic tumors will behave as if they were growing in a nonimmune animal. This resistance is said to be due to TSTA.

TAA specific to the tumor are thought not have any apparent role in this *in vivo* rejection process. Such antigens demonstrated in various *in vitro* systems are generally shared (or are said to be "cross reacting") among tumors which also show TSTA *in vivo*. In man, *in vitro* systems provide the only available tool and demonstrate only TAA; it is not surprising, therefore, that a high degree of "cross reactions" occur between various histogenetic types of tumors taken from different individuals.

The curious discrepancy between *in vivo* and *in vitro* behavior has no explanation which is widely accepted currently. No TSTA have been identified as cell surface molecules which are unequivocal targets for rejection and unique to the individual tumor. We are therefore limited in our considerations to antigenic structures present in tumor cell membranes which are associated with tumors, either exclusively or more frequently than in the analogous normal cell systems, and which can be demonstrated by available *in vitro* technics. Within this framework, however, a great deal has been learned about the variety and distribution of tumor-associated antigens in both animal and human models.

Tumor-associated antigens are generally but not exclusively confined to the cell surface membrane or its appendages. Among such antigens have been identified structures (a) resembling virus envelope proteins from onco-genic as well as nononcogenic viruses and endogenous leukemia viruses, (b) virus-associated structures which are not normally represented in the virus itself, (c) alloantigens associated with and indistinguishable from histocom-patibility antigens of certain types, and (d) fetal or embryonic structures apparently appropriate to early differentiation in fetal cell membranes but not normally found in the surface of a normal cell in significant quantities. In addition to these "time anomalous" structures, place or "organ anoma-lous" structures are occasionally found on tumors as well.

Even without the evidence to be presented here, there is ample reason to conclude from existing work that multiple immunogenic structures are presented in the tumor cell membrane, and which are capable of inducing an immune response. Only in tumors induced by specific oncogenic viruses (SV-40, polyoma, for example) can shared rejection target antigens be identified. In this situation, a high degree of "cross reactivity" in terms of tumor rejection is found *in vivo* between tumors induced by the same virus. These rejections appear to be based upon virus-specific structures present in the tumor membrane. These are therefore both TAA and TSTA. Such systems have obvious appeal to the immunologist who wishes to study *in vitro* structures and at the same time, analogous specific responding systems which have relevance to the rejection process.

During the past six years, we have developed a system for examining the character of, and response to, TAA in a system in which connective tissue sarcomas are induced inbred congenic mice by chemical carcinogens and in which there is no known oncogenic virus. The results of these studies has led to the concept that there are in such tumors multiple antigenic membrane proteins which evoke independent multiclonal responses in the tumor-bearing host.

The antigens in the system to be described are KC1 solublized membrane proteins derived from families of syngeneic tumors. These soluble tumor membrane preparations are employed in an *in vitro* system of which the measure is proliferation of lymphoid cells taken from tumor-immune or tumor-bearing hosts. Thus, the responsiveness of various subsets of lymphoid cells under a variety of conditions of tumor immunity, are assessed by a simple *in vitro* test. "Cross reactions" can be detected and quantitated using identical preparations from multiple syngeneic tumors on the same cell subsets.

These studies have established the antigenicity and immunogenicity of such preparations in terms of cell-mediated responsiveness and antibody binding *in vitro*. They are immunogenic when injected with appropriate adjuvants into a normal host, both in terms of inducing responsive lymphocyte and tumor-specific transplantation resistance to the homologous tumor. In the *in vitro* system, extensive shared responses between syngeneic nonhomologous tumor antigens have been found as would be expected from other studies. However, the temporal sequence of these responses are such as to suggest strongly that the immune host is responding to multiple antigens by the development of multiple clones of proliferating cells.

The character of the responding cells and the cell products is still under investigation but it apparently includes both T and B subpopulations and their subclasses and antibody of various classes. Progress has been made toward the identification of individual components of this complex mixture of tumor-associated membrane structures in terms of antigens. In this system, two and probably more of these structures are specific proteins which represent expression of the endogenous murine leukemia virus genome in the tumors themselves. These are the P15 and GP69-81 (GP-70).

MuLV proteins. The expression of these proteins and the density of their representation, when present, varies slightly among groups of syngeneic tumors according to available evidence. *In vitro* passage of the tumors which express these proteins augments individual MuLV protein expression. Antibodies raised to these MuLV proteins are widely represented in the sera of older mice from the same lines, indicating that the tumor membranes are probably not the only cell structures which can express endogenous virus in the normal host. These data generally support the concept of a multiplicity of antigenic determinants in chemically-induced tumor cell surfaces.

The data suggest the concept that the difference between the *in vivo* and *in vitro* behavior of chemical carcinogen-induced tumors may be a quantitative rather than a qualitative one. It is possible, at least, that the rejection of the critical mass of tumor cells, used to challenge tumor immunogenicity, requires a multipoint attack on membrane components. The homologous tumor would be the only one liikely to have the concatenation of responding lymphoid cell receptors necessary to recognize and to provide the intensity of attack required to prevent growth *in vivo*. Syngeneic tumors bearing another mix of the large number of possible membrane structures would likely induce a lesser number of corresponding subsets. Thus an insufficient number of points of membrane attack would be concentrated on the same critical tumor cell mass. It would be predicted from this hypothesis that quantitative differences in rejection behavior between the homologous and syngeneic tumors could be found insufficiently close in iron titrations. Data accumulated in this laboratory and that in the literature suggest that this is correct. A detail examination of the hypothesis will require better knowledge of the character of and separation of some of the membrane components of tumor cells in order to examine individual immunogenicity and the possibility that each in roles transplantation rejection *in vivo*. Such studies are underway.

II. The Prevalence of and Mechanism of Sustained Tumor Antigen Load

It is self-evident that, in order to provide initial and sustained antigenic stimulus to the host. The multiple antigenic structures of tumor cell membranes must reach appropriate cells and organs of the lymphoreticular system. On the other hand, the enormity of the tumor antigen load to which the system is subjected has only recently been appreciated. Evidence from multiple approaches indicates that in the circulation of the tumor-bearing individual are cells and individual clusters of tumor cells, tumor membrane proteins and peptides of tumor origin. This antigen load is apparently sustained as long as tumor is present and growing.

To illustrate the intensity of antigenic experiences in the tumor-bearing host, 23–35% of patients with carcinoma of the colon and breast have in one of five 5 ml peripheral blood samples, viable tumor cells or tumor cell clusters. Studies which are limited to venous blood draining the tumor area show an even higher occurance of living tumor cells. In animal systems, the tumor cells in venous or arterial blood can be enumerated more accurately. One study has shown up to 5,000,000 fibrosarcoma cells are released into the circulation per gram of tumor tissue per 24 hours.

At the cellular level, tumor membrane proteins have been detected by radioimmunoassay technics (fibrosarcomas) in mice and rat models and at least two human tumors—neuroblastoma and osteosarcoma. The carcinoembryonic antigen, a glycopeptide of entodermal tumor origin, has been measured to be as high as 1,000 nanograms per ml in patients with cancer of the colon. While these data do not establish sustained high level tumor antigen load in every circumstance, the evidence is strong that it is a major factor influencing the immunologic relationship between tumor and host.

III. Fate and Distribution of Tumor Antigen

The mechanism by which tumor antigens are released into the lymphatics and the circulation is usually assumed to be related to necrosis, or invasion of postcapillary venules or lymphatics. New evidence suggests, however, that many tumors spontaneously secrete tumor antigen as a consequence of rapid membrane turnover, both *in vivo* and *in vitro*. Tumor membrane proteins in large amounts are found in the supernatent of growing tumors *in vitro*—for example, methylcholantherene-induced fibrosarcomas and human neuroblastoma. Tumors which do not secrete large amounts of membrane turnover proteins may do so spontaneously in the immune host. Alexander and colleagues found that such tumors show low levels of secretion in the nonimmune host, but that these levels of membrane turnover antigens increase by orders of magnitude when the animal bearing the tumor is specifically sensitized. The relative importance and prevalence in animal and human tumors of spontaneous versus indirect membrane turnover secretion of tumor antigens is unknown at present and an important area for further investigation.

In conclusion, primary tumors and probably their metastases generate and contribute to high levels of circulating tumor cells and their membrane products. This continuous antigen load stimulates the immune response, but also has a major influence on the impact of this response in the tumor-bearing host.

IV. Tumor-Specific Immune Responses

Tumors in man and animal are resisted powerfully by the host elements of the host lymphoreticular system. Indirect evidence in morphologic studies has been available for many years wherein a strong correlation between the presence of lymphocytes, plasma cells and other cells comprising hypersensitivity-type reactions, occur around the growing tumors and in draining lymph nodes in cancer of the colon, breast, and the stomach. More recently, an additional degree of sophistication has been added to this type of analysis by demonstrations that favorable prognoses are associated with hypercellularity in the T and B cell regions of regional lymph nodes. Acellularity in these areas was associated with a bad prognosis. This indirect evidence of immunologic activity against tumors, while useful prognostically, did not establish immunologic resistance to tumor bearing.

More direct evidence comes with the classic experiments of Southam, et al., who injected intradermally into the original host suspended autologous tumor cells taken from terminally ill cancer patients. He observed that, despite the fact that the primary tumor was growing and ultimately would kill the patient, a high degree of resistance of growth or rejection of injected cells occurred up to levels approximating 10^5–10^6 tumor cells. Above this level, resistance could be overcome by increasing cell numbers. In animal systems, this clinical experiment has been conformed, establishing the specificity of the phenomenon with respect to TSTA, and providing evidence that cell-mediated immunity is invoked. Thus the tumor-bearing host can reject specifically autochthonous tumor cells, providing the inoculum of living cells is sufficiently small. The morphology of the rejection process is that of a delayed hypersensitivity reaction. This phenomenon appears to have considerable relevance to the nonoccurrance of distant metastatic spread of tumors, and provides a possible explanation of the marked descrepancy between the incidence of metastases in most tumors and the frequency of potentially metastatic cell clusters in the circulation.

The most compelling evidence for multicomponent immunologic responses to tumor antigen determinants comes from *in vitro* studies involving cell-mediated immunity and antibody. Cell-mediated immunity *in vitro* against tumor-specific or tumor-associated antigens is demonstrated by two different approaches. One involves interactions between lymphocytes and living tumor cells, the other is the lymphocyte response to tumor cell products. The most frequently employed assays involve mixing living tumor cells with large numbers of lymphocytes and assaying the end point of cell death or inhibition of tumor cell growth. In microcytotoxicity assays, the kinetics are complex and the problem of controls is formidable. Within the data generated, a population of normal peripheral blood cells taken from a tumor-bearing patient contains, from 1–3 per 300 lymphocytes, specifically cytotoxic for tumor cells. While the kinetics of the growth inhibition assay are even more difficult to interpret, a similar proportion of cells is apparently involved. Another end point assay in this approach involves interactions between tumor cell products and lymphokine (MIF, etc.) production by the reacting cells. This technic also demonstrates large proportions of cells which respond to the presence of tumor.

The second approach, of more recent vintage, involves avoidance of the use of cultured living tumor cells since these present multiple problems to the experimentalist. Solublized products of the tumor cell membranes have been obtained by various technics. These soluble products are used to stimulate proliferation in lymphoid cells or to bind to lymphoid cells, or to cause lymphokine production. Studies in this laboratory have emphasized this approach and will be described briefly.

Lymphocyte proliferation occurs regularly in the presence of potassium chloride solubilized tumor membranes derived from chemically-induced fibrosarcomas and from osteosarcoma in man. The kinetic patterns of this stimulation resembled closely that of T cell and B cell mitogens. The stimulation observed is, within limits, quantitative in reflecting the size of the responding subset of cells. It is specific in the sense which has been described in the first section of this paper wherein multiple specifications are documented.

Stimulation of lymphocytes is first demonstrated in the lymph nodes regional to the tumor early after inoculation of tumor and later it also occurs in spleen, nonregional lymph nodes, and peripheral blood cells. The timing of appearance of such responsive subsets as well as the multiplicity of specificities apparently recognized, suggests strongly that multiple subsets of lymphoid cells are involved. The class and subclass of lymphocytes stimulated in this assay have not been clearly defined as yet. Early regional lymph nodes do contain T cells stimulated by the antigen and, later, in all cell masses are cells sensitive to anti-immunoglobulin and complement. However, in the regional lymph nodes during most of the period of tumor bearing and later in the spleen there are large numbers of cells which are stimulated by the antigen but which are not reduced or destroyed either by pretreatment with anti-O or anti-Ig and complement. This suggests that a population of responsive "null" cells is present. This puzzling result invites further study.

From all *in vitro* studies it seems a reasonable conclusion that tumor bearing represents a state of extreme hypersensitivity in terms of the numbers of immunocompetent cells capable of responding to tumor antigen, providing the proper *in vitro* conditions are met. This strongly emphasizes the major paradox of tumor-specific immunity. That is, the host is hyperimmune in terms of the number and variety of cells which are capable of interacting with and killing the tumor *in vitro,* but this immunity is quite ineffective in relation to the primary or any other large tumor mass in the living host.

Cell-mediated immunity *in vivo* is also difficult to demc • trate in the mode of delayed hypersensitivity. That is, most of the patients with solid tumors fail to give evidence of dermal delayed hypersensitivity responses if injected with appropriate antigen derived from the tumor. Exceptions to this are in patients having malignant melanoma and a few other tumors. Tumor-immune mice who no longer bear the primary tumor easily demonstrate delayed dermal hypersensitivity reactions to tumor antigen in the ear or in the footpad; those with growing tumor give variable, mostly negative reaction. It would therefore appear that conditions associated with bearing a massive tumor load provide inhibitory influences which prevent both the elicited delayed hypersensitivity reaction and decreased effectiveness of cytotoxic cells in mediating tumor destruction.

V. Antibody-Mediated Immunity

Although it was thought earlier that solid tumors did not regularly stimulate specific antibody production, ample evidence has now accumulated that, providing the primary tumor is removed or the tumor load reduced drastically, antibodies specific to tumor cell determinants can be demonstrated by a number of different methods, including hemmaglutination, radioimmunoassay and other binding technics, complement fixation, and complement-mediated cytotoxicity. In the presence of tumor or recurrence of tumor, such antibody is often no longer measurable. Antibody against tumor-specific determinants has been shown to have markers of almost all subclasses of immunoglobulin for which search has been made; no specific prediliction for one class or another appears to exist in the tumor-bearing host.

It should be obvious that in the tumor-bearing individual having large amounts of circulating antigen, and circulating antibody, circulating antigen-antibody complexes should be expected. Antigen-antibody complexes have been demonstrated in most tumor-bearing individuals, and provide at least partial explanation for the failure to demonstrate antibody in the circulation of tumor-bearing individuals in earlier studies. Moreover, such complexes have major biologic consequences in terms of general effects on the host immune system and of specific effects on cell-mediated immunity.

The specific immune response to *non*tumor antigens appears also to be altered in the tumor-bearing host. This was first observed in clinical situations where it was found that delayed hypersensitivity responses to multiple naturally occurring bacterial and viral antigens were no longer demonstrable in some individuals with advanced tumors and particularly in those whose prognosis was poor. Moreover, when the responses of circulating lymphocytes of such individuals to such mitogens as PHA and Con A were examined; these were found to be reduced. This led to the conclusion that immunodeficiency occurs in the tumor-bearing host, and some even concluded that such immunodeficiency was a causative factor with respect to the development and fate of the tumor. This state of apparent immunodeficiency has been reexamined both in man and animal in recent past. Some studies from our laboratory appear to be pertinent.

In studies involving eight inbred, congenic lines of mice and over 40 transplanted and 20 primary fibrosarcomas, the secondary effects of tumor bearing were assayed during the entire course of the tumor-bearing episode. This was done by examining regional and nonregional nodes, spleen, thymus, peripheral blood, and bone marrow. The total mass of T and B cells in the various lymphoid cell mass was enumerated and related to various *in vitro* immunologic parameters. In summary, the data showed that the tumor-bearing animal was hyper-responsive to sheep erythrocytes as antigens in terms of the number of plaque-forming cells, had increased numbers of B and T cells (increased 2–5 fold) and that the mitogen responses of lymphocytes was increased appropriately. The only reduction found was in the numbers of T cells and the mitogen responses of T cells in the peripheral blood. Thus, tumor bearing in this model appears not to be suppressive but immunostimulatory. The effects of tumor-bearing resemble those of adjuvants, and suggest that the tumor-bearing individual is not immunologically incompetent. On the other hand, *in vivo* as well as *in vitro* studies show that the probable explanation for the absence of delayed hypersensitivity during periods of tumor bearing is related in part to circulating plasma factors, including perhaps antigen-antibody complexes. This effect is on the effector side of the delayed hypersensitivity reactions.

VI. Blocking and Other Immunosuppressive Effects Observed in the Tumor-Bearing Individual

A key observation in *in vitro* studies of cell-mediated immune responses to tumor cells or tumor cell products is that the responding cell population must be thoroughly freed of autologous patient or tumor-bearing animal serum in order to elicit colony inhibition or cytotoxicity responses. This suggested to Hellström that a factor in serum might be blocking or otherwise inhibiting cell-mediated immunity *in vivo*. In his important contribution, he showed that there is a factor in serum of 90–95% patients who have living, active tumors which inhibits cytotoxicity to the autologous tumor and to all tumors of related type. When the tumor was removed, the blocking factor disappeared; if the tumor recurred, blocking factor reappeared in the serum. The period required for disappearance is quite short—on the order of 2–7 days, depending upon the system examined and the type of tumor.

They found and we have confirmed, that blocking factor consists of a product of the tumor and a serum component. Their data showed that the specific inhibition was directed toward the lymphocyte and not the result of masking of tumor antigens. Others have now found blocking factors can be prepared artificially, using proper combinations between tumor specific antibody and solubulized tumor antigens. The most effective blocking effect occurs in combinations in slight antigen access. Blocking therefore gives an *in vitro* method for detecting the presence of circulating tumor antigen in the serum of tumor-bearing patients and animals. It moreover correlates closely with presence of living tumor and, therefore, with prognosis. Utilizing soluble tumor antigens as the stimulus for lymphocytes in the LPA system developed in this laboratory, we have also found that blocking factor can be easily detected and quantitated both in experimental tumors and in osteogenic sarcoma and neuroblastoma of man.

The full circle of evidence for blocking as a biologically significant phenomenon has been gained when serum containing such factors is infused into animals, which are then inoculated with the specific tumor. In comparison with controls, blocking factor increased the proportion of takes in experimental tumors.

In summary, blocking factor consists of either soluble tumor antigen or tumor antigen-antibody complexes. The specific antigen recognition capability of the responding lymphocyte is physiologically denuded of specific recognition receptors, thereby losing capacity to react to and effect tumor cell destruction *in vitro*. It is assumed, but not proven completely, that a similar mechanism operates *in vivo*. Tumor antigens or antigen-antibody complexes might compromise or ectopically trigger and inactivate potentially cytotoxic or cytostatic lymphoid cells and perhaps macrophages.

The term "unblocking factor" has been introduced into the literature by Sjögren and his colleagues. This refers to a phenomenon occurring when upon addition of serum from animals which have recovered from, or been cured of tumors, in an *in vitro* system, in which blocking is demonstrated, blocking is reversed or nullified. The best evidence to date suggests that such sera contain large amounts of free antibody which will bind the antigenic ligands responsible for the specific blocking effect at the lymphocyte cell-receptor level. An *in vivo* manifestation of this phenonomon has been shown in both polyoma and SV-40 virus-induced tumors of rats. The infusion of large amounts of unblocking sera apparently reduced tumor growth in these highly antigenic tumor systems. There is no evidence for such an effect in man as yet.

VII. Balanced State Concept

In summary, the tumor-host relationship seems to involve a balanced state between the reactive elements of the lymphoreticular system and the products of the tumor itself. The immune response is sufficient to control tumor growth in some respects, but in most cases insufficient to prevent its ultimate compromise of the animal or patient. A tentative synthesis explaining this paradox of hyperimmunity in the presence of growing tumor can be outlined briefly as follows.

A sufficient mass of tumor cells, probably critical for each tumor and host combination, secretes either spontaneously or under immunologic attack a continuous and large volume of membrane structures—the tumor-associated antigens of the tumor. Such antigens stimulate a multi-component immune response to the tumor and are continuously secreted thereafter into lymphatics and the circulation. This antigen load becomes a major factor in the tumor-host relationship. One can conceive concentration gradients in which the highest concentration of such tumor-generated components is in the immediate vicinity of the tumor. That is, it is in the intercellular fluid, in the draining lymphatics, and in the postcapillary venules through which most immunocompetent cells would approach the tumor. The tumor antigens immediately encounter antibody in the intercellular fluids and in the circulation and become "neutralized," producing circulating antigen-antibody complexes. This provides a vehicle by which immunocompetent cells bearing specific receptors for the tumor determinants may be ectopically triggered, modulated, or otherwise blocked, and thus unable to cope with the antigen gradient. Since blocking is a reversible process, reduction in antigen or complex concentration, perhaps as occurs in areas remote to the original tumor, results in restored responsiveness of cells and a mechanism for controlling metastases or concomitant immunity. Complexes probably also have secondary effects upon the effectiveness of macrophages in the expression or the effector side of delayed hypersensitivity responses. They probably also effect the mechanisms by which antibody-mediated lymphocytolysis occurs as well as direct T cell cytotoxicity. Thus, a steady state is established in which the primary tumor protects itself through a secretion gradient but at the same time the subthreshold numbers of tumor cells which escape from the primary and represent potential reported metastatic implants, are controlled by the immune mechanisms.

This oversimplified model requires much further verification, and doubtless modification, as new data are brought to bear on the issue. The implications, if correct, go directly to the heart of the accepted principle of treatment of cancer; it validates the doctrine that tumor load should be reduced to the lowest level possible by surgery, X-ray, and chemotherapy in order to produce the best results. The reduction in tumor antigen load may actually permit the elements of the hyperimmune patients' lymphoreticular system to control tumor cell micrometastases and potential metastatic spread, despite the fact that all tumor has not been removed. It is clear, therefore, that the surgeon, the radiotherapist, and the chemotherapist must learn to use powerful immunologic defense mechanisms more effectively.

BACKGROUND READING

Ankerst J, Steele G, Sjögren HO: Cancer Res 34: 1794, 1974.

Baldwin RW, Price MR, Robbins RA: Int J Cancer 11: 527, 1973.

Boyse EA, Old LJ: *In* Anfinsen CB, Potter M, Schechter AN (Eds): Current Research in Oncology. New York, Academic Press, 57–94, 1972.

Forbes JT, Nakao Y, Smith RT: J Exp Med (submitted).

Halliday WJ: J Immunol 106: 855, 1971.

Hellström I, Hellström KE, Sjögren HO, Werner GA: Int J Cancer 7: 1, 1971.

Kearney R, Nelson DS: Aust J Exp Biol Med Sci 51: 723, 1973.

Konda S, Nakao Y, Smith RT: Cancer Res 33: 2247, 1973.

Old LJ, Boyse EA, Clarke D, Carswell E: Ann NY Acad Sci 101: 80, 1962.

Prehn RT, Main JM: J Natl Cancer Inst 18: 769, 1957.

Smith RT: N Engl J Med 287: 439, 1972.

Smith RT, Forbes JT, Nakao Y, Konda S: *In* Lindahl-Kiessling K (Ed): Lymphocyte Recognition and Effector Mechanisms. Proc Eighth Leukocyte Culture Conference. New York, Academic Press, 1974.

Smith RT, Landy M (Eds): Immune Surveillance. New York, Academic Press, 1970.

Smith RT, Landy M (Eds): Immunobiology and the Tumor-Host Relationship. New York, Academic Press, 1975.

Theory of Allogeneic Reactivity and Its Relevance to the T-Cell Response to Normal and Oncogenic Cells

K. J. Lafferty, M.D.

Current immunologic theory postulates that immunocyte induction occurs when antigen binds to a specific receptor on the surface of a responsive cell. It may be important for this antigen to be presented to a responsive immunocyte on the surface of some other cell such as the macrophage. However, it is generally considered that this cell plays only a passive role in immune induction. In this presentation I would like to show that a stimulator cell is required for T-cell induction and moreover that this cell plays an *active role* in immune induction.

The Nature of Allogeneic Interactions

The idea that a stimulator cell is required for T-cell induction derives from a study of allogeneic interactions. The term allogeneic interactions covers those events involved in the interaction between immunocytes and allogeneic cells.

In its most simplified form, the basic interaction between two allogeneic cells can be written as follows:

$$S_{a^+} + R_{a^-} \rightarrow R'_{a^-}$$

Where S_{a^+} is a stimulator cell that expresses a particular factor a^+ and R_{a^-} is a responder cell that does not express the same factor, but expresses a complementary factor a^-. R'_{a^-} is the activated responder cell produced as a result of this interaction. This cell may undergo a number of division cycles leading to its further differentiation. A specific example of such a reaction would be the undirectional mixed leukocyte reaction (MLR).

From the Webb-Waring Lung Institute, University of Colorado Medical Center, Denver, Colo.

This work was supported by USPHS grants AI-03047 and CA 13419 and NSF grant GB 63219, and a fellowship from the International Union Against Cancer.

The conventional explanation of the basic allogeneic interaction is shown diagramatically in Figure 1. This explanation rests on three assumptions:

(1) R_a^- is an immunocyte (T-cell).

(2) a^+ is a cell surface antigen that can be recognized by antibody-like receptors (a^-) on the surface of R_a^-.

(3) The a^+/a^- interaction activates the responsive cell.

Thus, according to this concept, allogeneic interactions are immune responses initiated when the responsive T-cell makes contact with foreign histocompatibility antigen.

There is now a body of evidence indicating that this explanation of allogeneic interactions is inadequate. This evidence can be summarized as follows:

(1) Not all cells that carry foreign H-antigen will stimulate in allogeneic interactions. Stimulatory activity is a property confined to lymphoid cell populations; we use the term lymphoid to cover all mononuclear cells found in lymph, T-cells, B-cells and macrophages.

(2) Lymphoid cells lose their capacity to stimulate when their metabolic activity is inactivated, however such treatments do not affect their expression of H-antigen. Moreover cells inactivated with gluteraldehyde, which will not stimulate allogeneic T-cells, retain their capacity to bind specifically to the activated T-cell. Such evidence indicates that recognition and activation are not the same process. Thus the a^+/a^- interaction, while

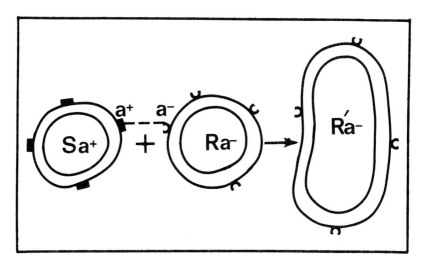

FIG. 1. Conventional explanation of interaction between a lymphocyte (Ra^-) and another allogeneic cell (Sa^+). Ra^- is an immunocyte carrying antibody receptors (a^-) for antigen (a^+) on the surface of the stimulator cell (Sa^+). $R'a^-$ is the activated responder cell produced as a result of this interaction.

it may be required for activation, is not a sufficient stimulus to cause the activation of the responsive cell.

(3) A further objection to the conventional explanation set out in Figure 1 concerns the nature of the responsive cell. While it is true that immunocytes respond in allogeneic interactions and produce specific effector cells as a result of their activation, the capacity to respond is not restricted to immunocytes. Thus immature blood cells devoid of immunocytes, such as the spleen cells of the chicken embryo, will also respond in allogeneic interactions.

In the light of all the above evidence we must reject the conventional concept of allogeneic interactions. In our view, the basic interaction,

$$S_{a^+} + R_{a^-} \rightarrow R'_{a^-}$$

must be considered in the following terms:

(1) The stimulator cell (S_{a^+}) is a *metabolically active* lymphoid cell (lymphocyte, macrophage); stimulation is an active and not a passive process.

(2) The responsive cell R_{a^-} is the hemopoietic stem cell or one of its more differential derivatives. Immunocompetent cells (T-cells) would be included among the derivatives of hemopoietic stem cells.

Relationship of Allogeneic Interactions to the Process of Normal Antigen Induction

There is no reason to assume that allogeneic reactivity had its evolutionary origin in a requirement for the blood cells of an animal to recognize and interact with those of another member of the same species. Thus, in considering these interactions we must assume that allogeneic reactivity is an abnormal expression of a normal physiologic function governing the interaction between cells of the lymphocyte-macrophage class and other blood cells. The Bretscher-Cohn theory of the way in which an immunocyte is tolerized or induced by antigen provides a conceptual basis which links allogeneic reactivity and normal antigen induction.

According to the Bretscher-Cohn theory, when antigen binds to an immunocyte, that cell receives "signal 1" (see Fig. 2). If the cell receives only "signal 1" it is tolerized. For induction of the immunocyte to occur, "signal 2" must be provided at about the same time as "signal 1." According to Bretscher and Cohn, "signal 2" is generated when antigen is simultaneously bound to the immunocyte's receptor and to associative antibody. We would modify this theory somewhat to suggest that "signal 2" is provided by a stimulator cell S which is bound to the responsive cell R by means of an antigen bridge (Fig. 2). The binding of the stimulator cell S to

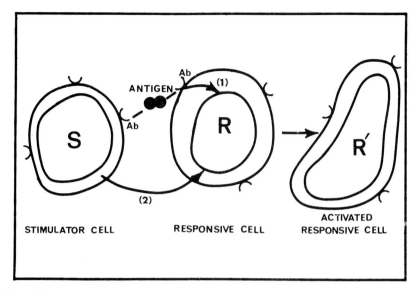

FIG. 2. Normal antigenic induction occurs when a responsive immunocyte R binds antigen to its surface receptor ("signal 1") and simultaneously receives an inductive stimulus ("signal 2") from a stimulator cell (S) which also carries antibody receptors on its surface. R' is the activated responsive cell.

the responsive cell R is controlled by receptors carried on the surface of S and R. In the case of the stimulator cell, this receptor may be the product of S, or could be a cytophylic product of some other cell.

Normal antigen induction now has the same general form as an allogeneic interaction. In both cases, induction depends not on a simple antigen-cell contact, but on the coming together of a stimulator cell and a responder cell. Antigen controls the specificity of the interaction but stimulation is an active function of the stimulator cell which provides "signal 2" for the responsive cell. We consider "signal 2" to be an inductive stimulus which causes the proliferation and further differentiation of the responsive cell.

In the following analysis of allogeneic interactions we will adhere to the two signal model for immunocyte induction. Our model will thus be based on the following postulates.

(1) Antigen binding to the immunocyte receptor delivers "signal 1." The delivery of "signal 1" alone is tolerogenic.

(2) Immunocyte induction only occurs when the responsive cell receives both "signal 1" and "signal 2."

(3) "Signal 2" is a nonspecific inductive stimulus provided by the stimulator cell.

(4) Immature blood cells respond to "signal 2" alone.

This last postulate is based on the following reasoning. We know empirically that immature blood cells respond in allogeneic interactions. Since these cells are not immunocytes they do not carry antigen-specific receptors and therefore cannot receive "signal 1." It follows therefore these cells must respond to "signal 2" alone.

Development of the Model for Allogeneic Interactions

Let us now return to the general statement of allogeneic interactions,

$$S_{a^+} + R_{a^-} \rightarrow R'_{a^-},$$

and consider the nature of the a^+/a^- interaction in terms of concrete examples. The most conservative assumption is that the a^+/a^- interaction represents the formation of an antigen antibody complex. According to such a model, the a^+ factor would be an antigen and the a^- factor would be an antibody that could combine with this antigen. We can now write the reactions for allogeneic interactions in two forms:

$$S_{ag} \times R_{ab} \xrightarrow[(2)]{(1)} R'_{ab} \qquad (1)$$

$$S_{ab} + R_{ag} \xrightarrow[(2)]{} R'_{ag} \qquad (2)$$

S is the stimulator cell (lymphocyte-macrophage) and R is a responsive cell which may be an immature blood cell or a T-cell. The two cells are brought together by the ag/ab interaction. In terms of cellular binding, the S_{ag}/R_{ab} interaction (reaction 1) will be equally as effective as the S_{ab}/R_{ag} interaction (reaction 2). That is, it is unimportant whether antibody recognition is mediated by the stimulator or responder cell. When the two cells come together, an opportunity will be provided for S to provide "signal 2" for the responsive cell. The bracketed figures indicate the signals received by the responsive cell. Thus we see that reaction 1 describes the allogeneic activation of T-cells (activated by signals 1 and 2) and reaction 2 describes the allogeneic activation of immature blood cells (activated by signal 2 alone).

We can specify this model more precisely in the following form,

$$S_{ag} + T_{ab} \xrightarrow[(2)]{(1)} T'_{ab} \qquad (3)$$

$$S_{ab} + {}^HR_{ag} \xrightarrow[(2)]{} {}^HR'_{ag} \qquad (4)$$

Reaction 3 describes the activation of T-cells (T_{ab}). This process can occur only when the responsive cell simultaneously receives "signal 1" and "signal 2." In such a case, the responsive cell must carry the ab receptor because "signal 1" is delivered only when antigen binds to a receptor on the surface of the responsive cell. Reaction 4 applies to the activation of immature blood cells ($^H R_{ag}$). These cells lack ab receptors by definition and are activated by "signal 2" alone. However to facilitate the surface interaction required for the passage of "signal 2," the stimulator cell must carry an ab receptor that can bind to ag on the surface of the responsive immature blood cell.

Phylogeny of Allogeneic Interactions

Allogeneic reactivity is not confined to members of the vertebrate phylum and any complete consideration of these reactions must attempt to integrate both vertebrate and invertebrate reactivity. Among the invertebrates, colonial ascidians (sea squirts) show allogeneic incompatibility reactions. These reactions prevent the stable fusion of incompatible colonies; when the cut surfaces of two incompatible colonies are placed together there is an initial fusion of the two vascular systems which is followed by a necrotizing reaction at the junction region. Allogeneic reactivity may be widespread among invertebrates; however, the genetics of these reactions have been studied only in the colonial ascidians. Such reactions are under the control of a single genetic locus which is polymorphic within the population.

We must now consider how we might relate invertebrate alloreactivity to the scheme outlined above, which so far as been developed within a framework of vertebrate type (antigen/antibody) recognition reactions; invertebrates, in general, do not possess an adaptive immune system of the type seen in vertebrates. The invertebrates may not pose a problem in this respect, but rather provide a solution to certain inadequacies of the theory so far developed. Vertebrate allogeneic interactions show both the adaptive character of the specific immune response and the nonadaptive species specific characteristic of ascidian alloreactivity. Adaptive responses are seen when one follows the generation of specific cytotoxic cells in mixed leukocyte culture (reaction 3). However cells other than immunocytes can also respond in allogeneic interactions (reaction 4), and in such cases the response does not result in the proliferation and differentiation of specific immunocytes. It is for this reason that these responses are not adaptive.

While our analysis of allogeneic interactions, which is summarized in reactions 3 and 4, provides an explanation for most of the known phenomena observed in mixed leukocyte reactions and in the graft versus host reactions, there are two examples of interactions of the reaction 4 class that are not readily explained if the interaction between the stimulator and the responder cell is mediated by an ag/ab interaction. These are the proliferative responses induced in the spleen of parental strain chicken embryos following the injection of adult F_1 hybrid blood leukocytes, and the capacity of irradiated adult F_1 animals to inhibit the growth of parental strain hemopoietic cells. In both cases the genetics of the situation preclude the involvement of ag/ab type recognition between the interacting cells.

Let us accept these problems as real difficulties for the theory based on the assumption that reaction 4 is mediated by ag/ab recognition reactions. If we assume that this nonadaptive component of the vertebrate response is a vestige of the type of alloreactivity observed amongst the invertebrates, we can press on with the analysis and examine what implications this assumption has for the vertebrate responses and how it would affect the relationship between vertebrate and invertebrate alloreactivity.

Oka's study of the genetics of ascidian alloreactivity suggests that genes controlling fusibility are the same as the genes that prevent self-fertilization. Fusion occurs between colonies of the same genetic constitution but fertilization does not. Within a given population, these fertility/fusibility genes are polymorphic; the population contains multiple alleles F_1, F_2 ---. The function of these genes, at least in the case of fertilization, is to prevent the intimate cellular cooperation of fertilization, a reaction involving both cytoplasmic and nuclear interactions. Thus the F factors may be considered as *inhibitors of intimate cellular interactions* (inhibitors for short). These factors control invertebrate alloreactivity and vertebrate analogues of these compatibility factors may also control nonadaptive vertebrate alloreactivity (reaction 4).

In such a situation, the delivery of "signal 2," thought to result from the cytoplasmic interaction between the stimulator and the responder cell, would be inhibited when the interacting cells are of the same genotype, but would be facilitated when cells differing at this locus come into contact. These interactions can be written as follows:

$$S^{F_1} + {}^H R^{F_1} \rightarrow \text{No interaction}$$

$$S^{F_2} + {}^H R^{F_1} \rightarrow {}^H R^{\prime F_1} \qquad (5)$$

Reaction 5 could represent invertebrate alloreactivity controlled by the F factors. A similar reaction could replace reaction 4 and describe the nonadaptive vertebrate response. In this case the controlling factors would be vertebrate analogues of the invertebrate F factors.

There is now a growing body of evidence that the most efficient S cell in vertebrate allogeneic interactions is the macrophage. The function of the F marker on the stimulator cell may be to allow this cell to signal other blood cells (inflammatory cells) when foreign agents have entered the organism, and to prevent such inflammatory responses under normal conditions. How could F factors exert this control in a system where both the stimulator and the responder carry the same F product (say F_1)? This could come about only if the binding of antigen to the stimulator cell in some way alters the phenotypic expression of its F factor. Antigen bound to or taken up by the S cell may interact with the surface F factor in such a way that the F_1 *antigen* complex is now phenotypically equivalent to F_2 or some other F factor. Such an event would release the stimulator cell from the restriction that forbids the activation of autologous cells, and such altered S cells would act as an inflammatory focus. The F factors are essentially acting as self-markers that prevent self-stimulation. Alteration of the self-marker releases the stimulator cell from this restriction. These reactions can be written in the following way,

$$S^A + {}^H R^A \rightarrow \text{No stimulation} \qquad (6)$$

$$S^A_{ag} + {}^H R^A \rightarrow {}^H R'^A \qquad (7)$$

where S^A is a stimulator cell carrying a self-marker of A genotype, ${}^H R^A$ is a potentially responsive immature blood cell carrying the same self-marker. S_{ag}^A is a stimulator cell carrying the A marker whose phenotype is altered by antigen (ag), and ${}^H R'^A$ is the activated cell produced in the interaction. Reaction 7 describes a nonspecific inflammatory reaction resulting from the alteration of the self-marker by antigen. Such a nonspecific inflammatory mechanism could operate in both vertebrate and nonvertebrate animals. It would be this type of blood cell activation that is responsible for the incompatibility observed when attempts are made to fuse tunicate colonies of different F genotype—that is, colonies carrying different self-markers.

The introduction of a self-marker concept into the control of S cell mediated activation of immature blood cells could have an influence on the specificity of the effector cells produced when vertebrate immunocytes are activated. If the formation of a self-marker-antigen complex is required to release the stimulator cell for the restriction that inhibits self-stimulation, then it is possible that the immunocyte receptor will not see just the antigen, but the self-marker-antigen complex. That is, the genotype of the stimulator cell will influence the specificity of the effector cell produced as a result of the interaction. In this context it is interesting to note that Shearer has shown that TNP modified spleen cells will generate specific cytotoxic cells (T-cells) when these cells are cultured with normal syngeneic spleen cells. However, the cytotoxic cells thus generated will lyse only TNP modified target cells of the same H-2 genotype as the stimulating cell population. Since there is no absolute requirement for both cytotoxic cells and traget cells to carry the same surface antigens (allogeneic killing is very efficient when an allogeneic cell is used to stimulate effector cell production), it would appear that the T-cells generated in Shearer's system are specific for the complex of TNP and a surface component of the stimulator cell. We

TABLE 1. Interactions between Stimulator Cells (S) and Immature Blood Cells ($^H R^A$) or T-Cells (T^A_{ab})

Identification	Interaction	Result	Comment
A	$S^A + {}^H R^A \longrightarrow neg.$	Zero	Normal resting situation in vertebrate and invertebrate animals
B	$S^A_{ag} + {}^H R^A \xrightarrow{(2)} R'^A$	Inflammatory response not antigen-specific	Reactivity seen in both vertebrate and invertebrate animals
C	$S^B + {}^H R^A \xrightarrow{(2)} {}^H R'^A$	Inflammatory response not antigen-specific	Allogeneic reactivity of both vertebrate and invertebrate animals
D	$S^A + T^A_{ab} \longrightarrow neg.$	Zero	Resting situation in immune system
E	$S^A_{ag} + T^A_{ab} \xrightarrow[(2)]{(1)} T'^A_{(Aag)}$	T-cell activation	Normal activation pathway in vertebrate animals
F	$S^B_b + \xrightarrow[(2)]{(1)} T'^A_{(Bb)}$	T-cell activation	Allogeneic activation of immune system in vertebrate animals

would suggest this complex is the self-marker-antigen complex. Thus we can write the reaction describing immunocyte induction in the following form,

$$S^A_{ag} + T^A_{ab} \xrightarrow[(2)]{(1)} T'^A_{(Aag)}$$

In this reaction $T'^A_{(Aag)}$ is an effector cell (T-cell) of A genotype which is specific for the Aag complex.

SUMMARY OF GENERAL MODEL

We have developed a general theoretical framework that interrelates inflammatory and allogeneic reactivity of both invertebrate and vertebrate animals. These antigen nonspecific responses form a mechanistic basis for the development of antigen specific immunocyte activation seen among the vertebrates.

We can summarize these ideas as follows:

(1) A self-marker system arose early in evolutionary development to prevent interaction between cells of like genotype. The self-markers are expressed on both germ cells of certain primitive organisms and are also expressed on the blood cells of both invertebrate and vertebrate animals.

(2) Inflammatory reactions are initiated when the self-marker carried by a stimulator cell (S) is modified by some foreign agent (antigen, ag). These modified S cells can then activate other blood cells and so set off the inflammatory response. This mechanism is essentially similar in both invertebrate and vertebrate animals and is described by reaction B in Table 1.

(3) Invertebrate alloreactivity occurs when blood cells carrying different self-markers interact (reaction C, Table 1). The resulting severe inflammatory response disrupts the vascular junctions and is seen as a rejection phenomenon.

(4) Vertebrate inflammatory reactions have an analogous mechanism to those of the invertebrates (2, above). One component of vertebrate allogeneic interactions (the activation of immature blood cells) is essentially the same as invertebrate alloreactivity (3 above).

(5) Vertebrate T-cells may be activated by either normal self-stimulation following modification of the self-marker by antigen (reaction E, Table 1). $T'^A_{(Aag)}$ is the resulting effector cell with specificity for the Aag complex. Vertebrate immunocytes may also be activated by allogeneic stimulation. In this case the stimulator and responder cell are of differing genotype and the foreign antigen (b) forms part of the surface of the S^B stimulator cell (reaction F, Table 1).

96 CANCER BIOLOGY, II

Application of Theory to the Transplantation Problem

Consider the situation where a tissue graft of B genotype is transplanted to an immunologically mature host of A genotype.

Events Occurring in the Transplant. Among the blood cells carried in the transplant (passenger leukocytes) one would expect to find responsive blood cells ($^{H}R^{B}$) which when activated by host stimulator cells (S) could set in motion an inflammatory reaction. Such a reaction would have the form,

$$S^{A} + {}^{H}R^{B} \xrightarrow{(2)} {}^{H}R'^{B} \quad (1)$$

This local inflammatory reaction in the transplanted tissue could damage the function of the allograft; such damage would be nonspecific.

Events Occurring in the Host's Immune System. The passenger leukocytes carried in the allograft will provide a source of stimulator cells of donor genotype ($S_{b}{}^{B}$), and these cells will carry the antigens (b) that are also expressed on the parenchymal cells of the transplant. These stimulator cells will interact with host T-cells and generate transplant specific cytotoxic cells. This reaction can be written,

$$S^{B}{}_{b} + T^{A}{}_{ab} \xrightarrow[(2)]{(1)} T'^{A}{}_{(Bb)} \quad (2)$$

Transplant derived antigen could also be presented to the host's T-cells via host stimulator cells. This reaction would have the form,

$$S^{A}{}_{b} + T^{A}{}_{ab} \xrightarrow[(2)]{(1)} T'^{A}{}_{(ab)} \quad (3)$$

It should be noted that the activated T-cells produced in this interaction would not be specific for the cells of the transplanted tissue. However T-cells of this class could act as helper cells for the production of antibody directed against the antigens (b) of the graft. Thus, reaction 3 could lead to the protection of the allograft by the production of humoral blocking factors.

The ultimate fate of an allograft will depend on the balance between those events leading to graft destruction and those tending to protect the graft from the host's cellular immune response. If reactions 1 and 2 dominate the protective effect of reaction 3, the graft will be destroyed. However, if the balance tilts in the opposite direction, the process of graft rejection will be curtailed. Since reactions 1 and 2 are dependent on the presence of passenger leukocytes in the grafted tissue, the complete removal of these elements from the transplant will enhance allograft survival.

It has recently been demonstrated that organ culture of thyroid tissue for an extended period—approximately 4 weeks—can greatly prolong the survival of such tissue when it is transplanted into an allogeneic recipient. During this culture period blood elements in the tissue die off but the parenchymal cells continue to express their transplantation antigens. This enhancement of allograft survival following organ culture can be attributed to a loss of passenger leukocytes from the transplanted tissue.

Application to the Tumor Situation

We now know that many tumors carry novel tumor-associated antigens, and that these antigens are often capable of activating the host's immune system. However, the response to these antigens will be determined, at least in part, by the nature of the cell that carries these antigens. The oncogenic change may occur in a cell that has stimulator characteristics. Such cells we might expect to be highly immunogenic and rapidly eliminated by the host's cellular immune response. Thus, tumors of this type are more likely to be seen when the host's immune system is impaired in some way, and it may be for this reason that reticulum cell sarcomas and lymphomas are relatively common among immunosuppressed individuals. Other tumors that do not have this intrinsic stimulator ability would have to activate the host's immune system indirectly, by way of the host's own stimulator cells. This process appears to activate both cytotoxic T-cells and helper T-cells, and in many cases the humoral blocking factors protect the tumor from the destructive effect of the cytotoxic cells.

Is there an immunologic solution to the tumor problem? At the moment we cannot answer this question. The hope is, that as we learn more about T-cell activation we may learn how to modulate the T-cell response to tumor antigens. What we must do is swing the balance of the immune response much more in favor of the cytotoxic cell response.

REFERENCES

1. Bach FH, Bach ML, Sondel PM, Sundharadas G: Transplant Rev 12: 30, 1972.
2. Croy BA, Osoba D: J Immunol 130: 1626, 1974.
3. Greineder DK, Rosenthal AS: J Immunol 114: 1541, 1975.
4. Helström KE, Helström I: Clin Immunobiol 2: 233, 1974.
5. Lafferty KJ, Walker KZ, Scollay RG, Killby VAA: Transplant Rev 12: 198, 1972.
6. Lafferty KJ, Cunningham AJ: Aust J Exp Biol Med Sci 53: 27, 1975.
7. Lafferty KJ, Cooley MA, Woolnough J, Walker KZ: Science 188: 259, 1975.
8. Oka H: In Profiles of Japanese Science and Scientists, Tokyo, Kodansha, 1970.
9. Shearer GM: Eur J Immunol 4: 527, 1974.

Postulated Relationships between Lysozyme and Immunoglobulins as Mediators of Macrophage and Plasma Cell Functions

Elliott F. Osserman, M.D.

The purpose of this paper is to review some of the evidence which indicates that lysozyme [1] is an important mediator of certain of the effector functions of macrophages and that the role of this enzyme may be comparable in importance to that of immunoglobulins in the effector functions of plasma cells. Some of the evidence which suggests a structural similarity between the active site of lysozyme and the combining site of immunoglobulins will also be indicated. In combination with the well documented physiologic interactions between macrophages and plasma cells, the possibility is raised that the more highly specialized and complex plasma cell-immunoglobulin systems may have evolved from and been patterned after the more primitive macrophage-lysozyme system.

It is obviously not possible to consider the interrelations between macrophages and plasma cells without also including T and B lymphocytes and their recognized functions. Table 1 presents an outline of macrophages, T and B lymphocytes and plasma cells, their specific functions and the presently recognized mediators of these functions. From the phylogenetic and evolutionary standpoints, it is noteworthy that the macrophage or "mononuclear phagocytic system" appears early in the evolution of lower order animals, whereas the more specialized T and B lymphocytic and plasmacytic systems appear much later in the vertebrates. Considered teleologically, it is not unexpected that the increasing structural complexity of the host would necessitate increasingly complex, versatile and specialized defense mechanisms. In this same framework, considerable interractions between and among these different cell types would be expected.

With respect to the macrophage or mononuclear phagocytic system, in

From the Institute of Cancer Research and Department of Medicine, College of Physicians and Surgeons of Columbia University, New York, N.Y.

These studies were supported by grant CA-02332 of the National Cancer Institute. The author is American Cancer Society Professor of Medicine.

TABLE 1. Cells of the Immune System, Their Functions and Mediators

Cell Type	Functions	Mediators
Macrophage —monocyte —mononuclear phagocyte system	Processing of particulate complex "macro-antigens" —"outside" bacteria fungi protozoa —"inside" membranes and cells-"self"	Enzymes lysozyme plasminogen activator acid hydrolases cathepsins peroxidase Complement components F_c (IgG) receptor
Lymphocytes T lymphocyte	Recognition	Receptor specific "Ig" type ? light chain
	Interactions with macrophages	"MIF," macrophage (migration) inhibitory factor "MAF," macrophage arming factor
	Effector delayed hypersensitivity graft vs. host cell-mediated cytotoxicity	"lymphokines"?? "toxins"??? interferon
	Modulation/regulation	"suppressor" ? RNA ? Ig
B lymphocyte ⎸ ⎸ ⎸ plasmacyte	Humoral defenses Modulation/blocking	Immunoglobulins IgG, IgA, IgM, IgD, IgE —complete (H_2L_2) —incomplete (L_2)

the higher vertebrates this system includes all tissue macrophages, alveolar macrophages, Kupffer cells and peritoneal macrophages, as well as circulating monocytes [2]. Present evidence indicates that there are several subpopulations of macrophages which are concerned with specific areas of defense, such as the lung, liver and peritoneum. The available evidence also indicates that there is little if any distant voyaging of these cells, i.e., the alveolar macrophages do not venture from the lung into the peritoneum, and vice versa. This specialization and compartmentalization is reflected in certain differences in the specific enzyme profiles of particular macrophage populations [3,4].

As indicated in Table 1, the principal function of macrophages is the processing of particulate and complex "macro-antigens." These include outside invaders, such as bacteria, fungi and protozoa but not most viruses. Of particular importance to our present consideration is the increasing evidence that macrophages are also involved in responses to endogenous "macro-antigens," particularly the membranes and organelles of cells under the conditions of neoplastic transformation [5].

The principal mediators of macrophage functions are apparently enzymes, and these can generally be grouped into externally-secreted enzymes which are released into the surrounding milieu, and internal-lysosomal enzymes which are retained within the cell and operate within the phago-lysosomal system. In Table 1, lysozyme is indicated as the principal secretory product of macrophages, and recent studies by Gordon and his associates [6] have indicated that macrophages produce and continuously release very large amounts of lysozyme. This synthesis is apparently independent of the physiologic state of these cells, in contrast to the synthesis of other enzymes such as collagenase [7] and elastase [8] which are dependent on macrophage stimulation. Thus, lysozyme must be considered a constitutive product of macrophages, presumably involved in the basic and major functions of these cells. It should be noted that lysozyme is also found in cells of the granulocytic series but, in contrast to macrophage lysozyme, granulocytic lysozyme is apparently restricted to the internal lysosomal setting, whereas in macrophages the enzyme is continuously released into the surrounding milieu. Plasminogen activator has also been shown to be another secretory product of macrophages. The physiologic significance of this enzyme is still undefined but it possibly functions under certain conditions in conjunction with lysozyme in the enzymatic degradation of complex membrane glycoproteins.

Macrophages also synthesize certain of the components of the complement system, and this capability, in conjunction with the presence on the surface of certain macrophages of a receptor for the Fc portion of IgG, enables the macrophage to interact with antibodies and participate extensively in antibody-dependent immune mechanisms. The chemical nature of the Fc receptor is presently unknown.

The internal-lysosomal enzymes of macrophages include the acid hydrolases,phosphatases, cathepsins, peroxidase, nuclease, lipases, etc. It is well established that these enzymes collaborate in the complex functions of digesting bacteria and other complex "outside" macro-antigens, i.e., processes which likewise involve the cleavage of complex proteins, polysaccharides, lipids and nucleic acids, Among the many key questions in this area which remain to be defined is the interrelationship between the cells of the monocyte-mononuclear phagocytic system and cells of the granulocytic series.

As stated previously, the T and B lymphocytic systems apparently evolved in response to the needs of higher order vertebrates for greater versatility and specificity of immune defenses. A detailed consideration of T cell functions is beyond the scope of this paper but it should be emphasized that the principal function of T cells appears to be the recognition and sensing of "foreignness." Substituting the terms "antigen" and "non-self" for "foreignness," T cells may be regarded as far-ranging "scouts" capable of penetrating remote tissue areas in the host in search of anything foreign. As yet, the precise biochemical mechanisms whereby this recognition is accomplished are unknown, but there is some evidence that T cells carry surface-specific macromolecules resembling immunoglobulins but perhaps limited to the hypervariable or combining-site regions of immunoglobulins. This hypothesis implies the presence of preformed antibody molecules consistent with Burnet's clonal selection theory.

T cells, having detected and recognized something foreign, respond by performing certain effector functions. The extent to which T cells differentiate into "effector" cells is still unclear and the specific mediators of T cell functions *per se* are still very poorly defined in biochemical terms. Even MIF, the macrophage inhibitory factor, whose physiologic functions have been relatively well delineated, is still minimally characterized biochemically. MIF is postulated to be a glycoprotein with a molecular weight in the range of 40,000, but beyond this, little is known of its molecular properties. For present considerations, however, MIF may be regarded as the signal released by T cells for the purpose of mobilizing and assembling regional macrophages to a specific site where "foreignness" has been detected. Again, teleologically, it would seem practical for the T cell "scout," which lacks much if not all of the enzymatic armamentarium needed to deal with an invader, to have the capability of summoning more adequately armed cohorts, i.e., the macrophages. T cells are also apparently capable of elaborating a specific macrophage-arming factor (MAF) as well as other lymphokines, toxins and interferon, but much of the evidence for these functions is still very incomplete.

From the evolutionary and phylogenetic standpoints, the development of a population of cells with the function of synthesizing and releasing specific protective molecules, i.e., immunoglobulins, is certainly the most recent and, therefore, the most sophisticated and specialized immunoligic capacity. Stated differently, the more basic macrophage products are enzymes operative against *classes* of compounds, e.g., carbohydrates, proteins and lipids, as opposed to immunoglobulins which are interactive with *only certain* proteins, carbohydrates, etc., having specific molecular configurations. Rephrasing the earlier thesis, increasingly specific and selective molecules have been evolved to serve the needs for greater specificity in structurally complex hosts.

B lymphocytes are characterized by the presence of surface immunoglobulins. When in contact with specific antigens, B cells multiply and differentiate into cells which release immunoglobulin, and these "secretory" B cells are apparently the same as plasma cells. Much of our present information concerning the detailed structure and function of immunoglobulins has been derived from analyses of Bence Jones proteins and serum immunoglobulins associated with multiple myeloma and related plasma cell dyscrasias [9–11]. We now recognize five major classes of immunoglobulins, IgG, IgM, IgA, IgD and IgE, with structurally distinct heavy chains (γ, v, α, and ϵ), and two structurally distinct types of light chains, designated κ and λ, respectively. The combination of limited sections, i.e., the hypervariable regions of both the light and heavy chains, makes up the specific antibody-combining site of each immunoglobulin. Recent evidence suggests that some, if not all, antibodies may possess more than one specificity and thus have the capacity to bind structurally different haptens in different parts of the combining site [12]. If this proves a general characteristic of antibodies, it would imply the need for fewer individual immunoglobulins to provide the spectrum of antibody specificities found in higher animals.

Recent crystallographic analyses [13,14] of a small number of human and mouse myeloma proteins which exhibit some combining ("antibody") activity have provided more detailed information on the dimensions and contours of antibody-combining sites and how these are derived from the specific amino acid residues of the heavy and light chains. Although a detailed review of these data is beyond the scope of this paper, it has been clearly established that the combining site is a hydrophobic pocket or cleft, with dimensions comparable to those of the active site of the lysozyme molecule [15,16]. It is noteworthy that Phillips, who was primarily responsible for elucidating the structure of hen egg-white lysozyme, and Porter, who pioneered in determining the subunit structure of immunoglobulins, both anticipated several years ago that this structural similarity between lysozyme and immunoglobulins might exist [17,18].

Functions of Lysozyme—Known and Postulated

Whereas immunoglobulins are restricted to higher order vertebrates, lysozyme, at least in the generic sense, is virtually ubiquitous throughout nature [reviewed in reference 1]. Thus, enzymes capable of cleaving complex polysaccharides by the hydrolysis of β-1,4 glucosidic linkages are to be found throughout the vertebrate and invertebrate animal kingdom, as well as in plants, bacteria, fungi and even viruses. Again considered teleologically, the cleavage of complex polysaccharides is unquestionably critical for both the development and defense of living organisms. Nature appears to have evolved a basic molecular pattern for accomplishing these functions and adapted, amplified and modified this basic pattern in many and diverse ways for specific needs in specific settings.

Unquestionably, the most extensively studied and best delineated function of lysozyme is that initially discerned by Fleming, i.e., its bacteriolytic action [19], and particularly within the lysosomal setting of the granulocyte, lysozyme's function would appear to be primarily, if not exclusively, antibacterial. Likewise, the lysozyme in tears and secretions of the respiratory and intestinal tracts might also be reasoned to be principally antibacterial. Macrophage lysozyme unquestionably also serves antibacterial functions, probably in conjunction with complement and antibody, but the rapid release of the enzyme would suggest that it may participate in some of the nonphagocytic functions of macrophages, possibly including functions pertaining to immune and nonimmune surveillance of host membranes related to neoplastic transformation. The evident importance of macrophages in antitumor defenses, together with demonstrated abundance of lysozyme synthesis by these cells, would seem to make this a reasonable hypothesis deserving critical investigation.

Efforts in our own laboratory over the past few years have been focused on determining whether lysozyme has any significant effects on mammalian cells and their constituent organelles and membrane macromolecules. We were initially led to this line of investigation by our observation that very large quantities of lysozyme were present in the serum and urine of patients with monocytic and monomyelocytic leukemia [20]. We made this observation initially on a patient with plasma cell myeloma whose - course terminated in acute monocytic leukemia. This, parenthetically, is again illustrative of the major functional interrelationship between the plasmacytic and monocyte-macrophage systems. It was subsequently demonstrated that both mice [21] and rats [22] with monomyelocytic leukemia also elaborated large quantities of lysozyme, and this has enabled the purification and detailed biochemical characterization of these mammalian lysozymes as well as the investigation of their effects on cells, organelles and membrane components. In our initial studies, we investigated the effects of lysozyme on normal and transformed mammalian cells in tissue culture [23]. With normal and SV40 transformed mouse 3T3 cells, lysozyme produced a relatively small and transient inhibition of both proliferation and uptake of H_3 thymidine. These effects were particularly evident when lysozyme was incorporated in the medium from the time of initiation of cultures, and there was significantly less effect when the enzyme was added after 48 hours *in vitro*. The qualitative effects of lysozyme on the pattern of *in vitro* growth of mouse embryo fibroblasts were even more striking than its effects on cell proliferation and thymidine uptake. Thus, SV-3T3 cells grown in the presence of lysozyme showed a more uniform monolayer pattern, suggesting a reacquisition of contact inhibition.

The effects of rat and hu nan lysozyme were also studied on spontaneously transformed rat liver cells. Again, very striking cytologic alterations were observed, consisting mainly of a flattening of cells and the appearances of extensive cytoplasmic projections which were particularly well demonstrated by scanning electron microscopy [23]. In more recent studies [24], we have observed a change in the pattern of growth and clonal morphology of H5-J11 cultured Novikoff hepatoma cells. Colonies of these cells grown in the presence of lysozyme exhibit a more diffuse and dispersed pattern compared with a more dense clonal architecture in control cultures.

Recently Asdourian et al. [25] have reported that hen egg-white lysozyme modifies the morphology of cultured chick embryo cells from stellate to elongated spindle-shaped forms without altering protein or nucleic acid synthesis. They also found that lysozyme increased the rate of glucose uptake and decreased the ConA binding of both chick embryo and HeLa cells. Lysozyme treatment of hexosamine-labeled monolayers resulted in the release of hexosamine in a TCA-soluble fraction. These effects could be inhibited by anti-lysozyme antiserum and/or the trisaccharide of N-acetylglucosamine, and were not duplicated by protamine, insulin or bovine serum albumin. These results are apparently consistent with our observations using mammalian cells and mammalian lysozymes [23,24] and provide additional evidence that lysozyme has significant effects on the structure and function of animal cells. Now that these actions of lysozyme have been demonstrated, the specific lysozyme substrate lysozyme in animal cells must be identified, and the physiologic and pathologic significance of these lysozyme activities must be defined.

Summary

The general pattern of organization of the "macrophage-lysozyme" and "plasma cell-immunoglobulin" systems has been reviewed, along with some of the evidence that lysozyme is an important mediator of certain of the effector functions of macrophages. In addition to its bacteriolytic actions, macrophage lysozyme may have functions related to host cells and their constituent membranes and organelles. The possible physiologic significance of these lysozyme actions is considered.

REFERENCES

1. The chemistry and physiology of lysozyme are reviewed in detail in: Osserman EF, Canfield RE, Beychok S (Eds): Lysozyme. New York, Academic Press, 1974.
2. Edited by van Furth R (Ed): Mononuclear Phagocytes. Oxford and Edinburgh, Blackwell Scientific Publications, 1970, pp 654.
3. Myrvik QN, Leake ES, Fariss B: J Immunol 86: 133, 1961.
4. Cohn ZA, Wiener E: J Exp Med 118: 991, 1963.
5. Evans R, Alexander P: Immunology 23: 615 and 627, 1972.
6. Gordon S, Todd J, Cohn ZA: J Exp Med 139: 1228, 1974.
7. Werb Z, Gordon S: J Exp Med 142: 346, 1975.
8. Werb Z, Gordon S: J Exp Med 142: 361, 1975.
9. Kochwa S, Kunkel HG (Eds): Immunoglobulins. Ann NY Acad Sci 190: 584, 1971.
10. Kabat EA: General features of antibody molecules. Presented at 3rd Int. Convoc. Immunol., Buffalo, N.Y., 1972. Specific Receptors of Antibodies, Antigens and Cells. Basel, Karger, 1973, pp 4–30.
11. Osserman EF, Takatsuki K, Farhangi M, et al: Plasma cell dyscrasias: general considerations, plasma cell myeloma: primary macroglobulinemia; amyloidosis; heavy chain diseases. In Williams WJ, et al (Eds): Hematology. New York, McGraw-Hill, 1972, pp 950–984.
12. Richards FF, Konigsberg WH, Rosenstein RW, Varga JM: Science 187: 130, 1975.
13. Poljak RJ, Amzel LM, Avey HP, et al: Proc Natl Acad Sci USA 70: 3305, 1973.
14. Padlan EA, Davies DR: Proc Natl Acad Sci USA 72: 819, 1975.
15. Phillips DC: Proc Natl Acad Sci USA 57: 484, 1967.
16. Phillips DC: Sci Am 215: 78, 1966.
17. Phillips DC: Harvey Lect 66: 135, 1972.
18. Porter RR: Harvey Lect 65: 157, 1971.
19. .Fleming A: Proc Roy Soc, Ser B 93: 306, 1922.
20. Osserman EF, Lawlor DP: J Exp Med 124: 921, 1966.
21. Warner N, Moore MAS, Metcalf D: J Natl Cancer Inst 43: 963, 1969.
22. Rosenthal DS, Moloney WC: Proc Soc Exp Biol Med 126: 682, 1967.
23. Osserman EF, Klockars M, Halper J, Fischel RE: Nature 243: 331, 1973.
24. Qunicy DA, Osserman EF: Fed Proc 3: No. 3, Abstract 288, 1975.
25. Asdourian H, Chu L, Lau K, Amos H: Biochem Biophys Res Commun 64: 1142, 1975.

Molecular Events in Chemical Carcinogenesis

I. Bernard Weinstein, M.D.

Recent estimates based on epidemiologic data indicate that approximately 80% of human cancer is due to environmental, rather than inborn or genetic, factors. In addition, the evidence from occupational exposure, the association of cigarette smoking with lung and bladder cancer and the increasing association of other human cancers with exposure to specific chemicals and drugs indicate that the major environmental factors responsible for cancer causation are chemical agents rather than viruses. This does not, of course, deny the possibility that viruses or viral-related genes may play a role in the mechanism by which a normal cell is transformed to a cancer cell by chemicals, and I will return to this aspect later. Nevertheless the epidemiologic data suggest that identification and removal from our environment of the more potent chemical carcinogens could lead to a marked decrease in cancer incidence and mortality.

This year marks the bicentennial of the discovery of the first cause of cancer. It was in 1775 that the English physician Sir Percival Pott published a small book on his Chirurgical Observations in which he provided an explanation for why young men employed at that time as chimney sweeps developed cancer of the skin of the scrotum. Pott reasoned that "the disease, in these people, seems to derive its origin from a lodgement of soot in the rugae of the scrotum." This astounding "break-through" in cancer causation went largely unrecognized for more than a century. About 150 years later Kennaway and his colleagues demonstrated that the major carcinogenic agents in soots and coal tars were benzo(a)pyrene and related polycyclic aromatic hydrocarbons. We now know of at least 30 compounds that are carcinogenic in the human, and a partial list of these is given in Table 1. It is important to emphasize the extreme diversity of their structures. This aspect considerably complicates the problem of carcinogen detection, identification, and bioassay, as well as attempts to formulate a general theory of the mechanism of chemical carcinogenesis. Some of the

From the Institute of Cancer Research, College of Physicians and Surgeons of Columbia University, New York, N.Y.

TABLE 1. Chemicals Recognized as Carcinogens in Humans

Chemical	Site of Cancers
Chemical mixtures	
Soots, tars, oils	Skin, lungs
Cigarette smoke	Lungs
Industrial chemicals	
2-Naphthylamine	Urinary bladder
Benzidine	Urinary bladder
4-Aminobiphenyl	Urinary bladder
Chloromethyl methyl ether	Lungs
Nickel compounds	Lungs, nasal sinuses
Chromium compounds	Lungs
Asbestos	Lungs
Arsenic compounds	Skin, lungs
Vinyl chloride	Liver
Drugs	
N,N-bis(2-chloroethyl)- 2-naphthylamine	Urinary bladder
Bis(2-chloroethyl)sulfide (mustard gas)	Lungs
Diethylstilbestrol	Vagina
Phenacetin	Renal pelvis
The Pill	Benign hepatomas
Naturally occurring compounds	
Betal nuts	Buccal mucosa
Aflatoxins	Liver
Potent carcinogens in animals to which human populations are exposed	
Sterigmatocystin	Liver
Cycasin	Liver
Safrole	Liver
Pyrrolizidine alkaloids	Liver
Nitroso compounds	Esophagus, liver, kidney, stomach

(Modified from Heidelberger C: Ann Rev Biochem, pp 79–121, 1975).

compounds listed in Table 1, e.g., benzidine, nickel, asbestos and vinyl chloride, represent occupational hazards. Others are drugs used in clinical practice, an example of which is diethylstilbesterol, which acts transplacentally as a carcinogen in humans.

Table 2 lists the major biologic facts pertaining to chemical (and in certain cases to radiation) carcinogenesis. In terms of human exposure it is important to stress the apparent lack of a threshold dose and the long lag

TABLE 2. Chemical Carcinogens—Basic Biologic Facts

1. Carcinogenesis is *dose dependent*—the larger the dose the greater the incidence of tumors and the shorter the lag. There is no evidence of *a threshold dose* below which a carcinogen is safe.
2. There is a *long lag* between exposure and the appearance of tumors. In humans this is about 5–30 years. In various species the lag is generally proportional to the lifespan of the species. Carcinogens can act transplacentally, with tumors appearing only later in the adult progeny.
3. Conversion of a normal tissue to a malignant neoplasm is a *multistep process*.
4. The action of certain types of carcinogens, so-called *initiating agents,* is markedly enhanced by *promoting agents, hormonal agents* and various *cofactors*.
5. Cellular *proliferation enhances* carcinogenesis.
6. Neoplasms induced by the same chemical carcinogen often display *antigenic diversity,* as well as a general *diversity of phenotypes* in terms of growth rate, degree of differentiation, cell surface properties, enzyme profiles, etc.

between exposure and the appearance of tumors. In terms of our eventual understanding of the mechanisms(s) underlying chemical carcinogenesis, the multistep nature of the process, the contribution of promoting agents and other cofactors, and the diversity of the phenotypes of individual tumors produced by a pure carcinogen in the same tissue, are all properties that can not be ignored.

A considerable amount of information has been obtained in the past 20–30 years on the metabolism of carcinogens by cells and on the initial interactions between carcinogens, or their metabolites, with specific cellular targets. The essential findings are listed in Table 3.

Largely due to the work of James and Elisabeth Miller, we now know that many chemical carcinogens undergo metabolic activation *in vivo* to form electrophilic reactants that bind covalently to cellular macromolecules including proteins, DNA and RNA. This is one of the few unifying principles in this field. At the present time it is not clear which (if any) of these targets is the critical one in terms of the process of cell transformation. It seems likely, however, that covalent binding is essential for the action of many, but probably not all, carcinogens since experimental maneuvers that prevent or reduce covalent binding generally inhibit carcinogenesis. An example of the complexities of metabolic activation of a carcinogen and the interaction of competing pathways of detoxification and conjugation are shown in Figure 1. The example illustrates how species and tissue specific metabolic factors, as well as exogenous factors, influence the extent to which a potential carcinogen becomes bound to cellular macromolecules.

Although covalent binding appears to be a necessary condition for the action of numerous carcinogens, it is not a sufficient condition, since covalent binding to macromolecules can often be detected in tissue in addition to those in which tumors are induced. The other determinants required for tumor induction have not been elucidated with certainty, although DNA repair, cell proliferation and promoting factors are frequently invoked.

Within the past few years, important information has also been obtained on the early effects that carcinogens exert on macromolecular synthesis in the target tissues. The major findings are listed in Table 4.

An extremely important area of carcinogenesis is that related to DNA repair. It is known that a variety of carcinogens induce unscheduled DNA synthesis or so-called excision repair, as well as single and double stranded DNA breakage. Direct chain scission may occur as an effect of x-rays or depurination. Enzymatic excision of "bulky lesions," i.e., those due to UV-induced thymine dimers, AAF, benzo(a)pyrene, and 4NQO are apparently mediated by a specific endonuclease which appears to be deficient in certain patients with the hereditary disease xeroderma pigmentosa. The later finding as well as recent studies from Setlow's laboratory on the effects of UV radiation and photoreactivation on tumor induction in fish provide indirect evidence that DNA may be a critical target during radiation or chemical carcinogenesis. Recent studies by Goth and Rajewsky (Proc Natl Acad Sci USA 71: 639, 1974) indicate that the extent of O-6 alkylation of guanine by

TABLE 3. Chemical Carcinogens—Basic Biochemical Facts

1. They include both man-made and natural products that have extremely diverse chemical structures.
2. They are subject to both metabolic activation and detoxification *in vivo*.
3. The metabolically activated forms are highly reactive electrophiles that bind covalently to nucleophilic residues in cellular proteins and nucleic acids.
4. The binding to protein is quantitatively greater than binding to nucleic acids and has a specific activity of about 1 residue of carcinogen/10^3–10^4 amino acid residues. The amino acid residues are usually the S of methionine or cysteine, N-1 of histidine or C-3 of tyrosine. Numerous proteins are attacked, both nuclear and cytoplasmic, although a few proteins (example, the "h_2"), whose specific function(s) are not known, are preferential targets.
5. Both RNA and DNA are targets and the specific activity is about 1 residue of carcinogen/10^4–10^5 nucleoside residues. Most carcinogens bind preferentially to guanine, but adenine and cytosine are also targets.
6. The binding to DNA is fairly random in terms of gene specificity. Both main band and satellite DNA are involved, as is mitochondrial DNA. There is some evidence for crosslinking.
7. The binding to RNA appears to involve all species of RNA; tRNA often has a higher specific activity than rRNA.

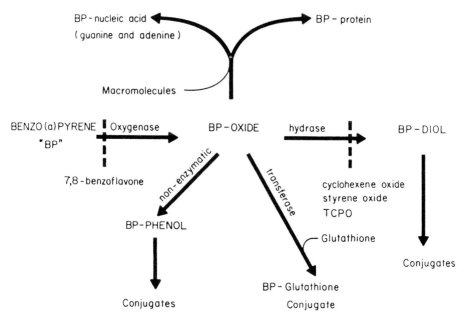

FIG. 1. Proposed scheme of microsomal metabolism of BP, leading to various detoxification products and to nucleic acid binding. BP-protein and BP-nucleic acid designate the reaction products of BP with protein and nucleic acid, respectively. ----, apparent sites of action of the various inhibitors. (For additional details see Pietropaolo and Weinstein: Cancer Res 35: 2191–2198, 1975; reproduced by permission.)

TABLE 4. Chemical Carcinogens—Early Effects on Macromolecular Synthesis

---

1. *Replication.* The binding to DNA induces unscheduled DNA synthesis (excision repair), single- and double-stranded DNA breakage. Most but not all carcinogens are mutagens. They can induce errors in base pairing, frame shift errors, deletions, and chromosomal breakage.
2. *Transcription.* There is an early inhibition of RNA synthesis which is somewhat preferential for the 45s ribosomal RNA precursor. Effects on RNA processing have not been studied extensively.
3. *Translation.* There is often an early inhibition of protein synthesis associated with release of ribosomes bound to the endoplasmic reticulum and disaggregation of polysomes. Function of carcinogen-modified tRNA or mRNA is inhibited.
4. *Regulation.* Enzyme induction (tyrosine aminotransferase) may be blocked. The pattern of transcription is altered—fetal genes depressed, etc. Effects on chromatin structure and function remain to be elucidated. Latent oncornaviruses frequently may be activated.

---

ethylnitroso-urea and the efficiency of removal of that lesion from cellular DNA are important determinants in the induction of central nervous system tumors. On the other hand N-7 alkylation of guanine, even though it occurs to a quantitatively greater extent than O-6 alkylation, does not appear to correlate with carcinogenicity. Similar evidence has been obtained by Anthony Pegg with dimethylnitrosamine-induced kidney tumors. These studies suggest the importance of specific types of alkylated bases in DNA in terms of the process of carcinogenesis.

Although there has been a tendency to emphasize the binding to DNA and the mutagenic activity of these agents, it is apparent from Tables 3 and 4 that carcinogens attack other cellular macromolecules and exert effects on macromolecular synthesis not only at the level of DNA replication but also at the levels of gene transcription and translation. Personally, I believe that the effects of carcinogens on the control of gene expression may turn out to be more important than their mutagenic effects, and this aspect deserved further intensive study.

As indicated above, it is now an axiom in cancer biology that many chemical carcinogens bind covalently to cellular nucleic acids. A logical question which follows is whether this binding produces detectable changes in the physical structure and functional properties of the modified nucleic acids. For the past several years our laboratory has been engaged in studying this aspect of chemical carcinogenesis and I will now briefly review our results.

Most of our studies have been with the potent liver carcinogen N-2-acetylaminofluorene (AAF). We have taken advantage of the important discovery in the laboratory of James and Elizabeth Miller that both RNA and DNA will react nonenzymatically *in vitro* with the N-acetoxy derivative of AAF. The major product obtained from hydrolysates of the modified nucleic acids is 8-(N-2-fluorenyl-acetamido)-guanosine which is the same derivative as that obtained following *in vivo* administration of the parent compound. The attack by AAF on the C-8 position of guanosine residues does not directly interfere with the hydrogen bonding involved in base pairing between guanosine and cytosine residues, and yet we could readily demonstrate impairment in the functional properties of AAF-modified tRNA or synthetic condons. This led us to hypothesize that binding of the bulky AAF molecule is associated with a conformational change in the modified nucleic acid. This was confirmed in molecular model building studies and analysis of the physical properties of AAF-containing dinucleoside monophosphates. On the basis of these and related studies we proposed a specific 3-dimensional conformation for nucleic acids at sites of AAF modification which we have named "base displacement."

The Base Displacement Model

In nucleic acids with Watson-Crick geometry the deoxyribose (or ribose) residues occupy a position with respect to the base residue referred to as "Anti." In the Anti conformation there is considerable crowding at the C-8 position of purine residues. We predicted, therefore, that attachment of the bulky AAF residue requires a rotation of about 180° of the guanine moiety around the glycosidic (N_9-C_1) bond to a position referred to as "Syn." Similar conclusions were reached by Kapuler and Michelson based on studies with guanosine residues modified by either Br or AAF at the C-8 position. Computer display studies and circular dichroism (CD) and proton magnetic resonance (pmr) data obtained with AAF modified oligonucleotides suggested additional conformational changes and led to the specific structure we refer to as "base displacement". This model is depicted in Figure 2. In addition to the Anti to Syn change, the modified guanine residue is displaced from its normal coplanar relation with adjacent bases. The fluroene residue occupies the former position of the displaced guanine and the fluorene is therefore stacked coplanar to an adjacent base. Strong evidence for this stacking interaction was provided by the CD and pmr studies of AAF modified oligonucleotides.

Extensive studies of the physical structure of AAF-modified double

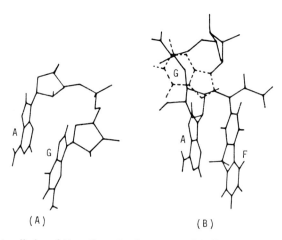

(A)   (B)

FIG. 2. Computer display of three-dimensional structure of ApG and ApG-AAF. (A) The conformation of ApG with Watson-Crick type geometry. (B) The base displacement model of ApG-AAF. The fluorene and adenine rings are stacked with optimum overlap and the displaced guanine is represented by dashed lines. In the figure "A" designates the adenine, "G" the guanine and "F" the fluorene rings. (For additional details see Nelson et al: J Mol Biol 62: 331–346, 1971; reproduced by permission.)

TABLE 5. Predictions of the Base Displacement Model

---

1. AAF modification *inactivates* the base pairing capacity of the modified guanine residues. It should produce mainly frame shift or deletion mutations rather than base substitution mutations.
2. The structural and functional changes induced in nucleic acids by AAF are in part a function of the bases neighboring the modified guanine residue.
3. AAF preferentially attacks guanine residues present in single-stranded regions of nucleic acids. Stabilization of double-stranded regions by ionic factors or protein binding should decrease their susceptibility to attack by AAF.
4. AAF modification of double-stranded DNA or RNA produces localized regions of denaturation.
5. In addition to AAF, the base displacement model may apply to other polycyclic aromatic hydrocarbon carcinogens that bind covalently to nucleic acids.

---

stranded DNA are also consistent with the base displacement model and a computer display of double stranded DNA containing an AAF modified G residue in the base displacement position indicates that the fluorene residue can be accommodated within the structure by disruption of the related G-C base pair.

The base displacement model makes several predictions and these are listed in Table 5. Each of these predictions has now been verified by extensive studies on the physical and functional properties of AAF modified oligonucleotides as well as high molecular weight RNAs and DNAs. This evidence has been summarized in recent review articles (Weinstein and Grunberger, 1974; Weinstein, Grunberger and Blobstein, 1974; Grunberger and Weinstein, 1975).

The results are of interest from a biologic point of view for two reasons: (1) They indicate that a carcinogen has a certain degree of specificity in terms of its attack on specific regions of nucleic acids and (2) That the structural changes induced by this attack are in part a function of the base sequence and the secondary and tertiary structure of the nucleic acid in the region of the nucleic acid which undergoes modification. It is likely that *in vivo* the quarternary structure of nucleic acids, i.e., their organization with proteins, is also an important factor. This could be of considerable importance in terms of the organization of DNA within the complex structure of cellular chromatin and in current studies we are addressing ourselves to this problem.

Figure 3(A) contrasts intercalation, of the type described by Lerman for planar compounds that bind non-covalently to nucleic acids, to the base displacement model which I believe may apply not only to AAF but also to other polycyclic aromatic carcinogens that bind covalently to nucleic acids.

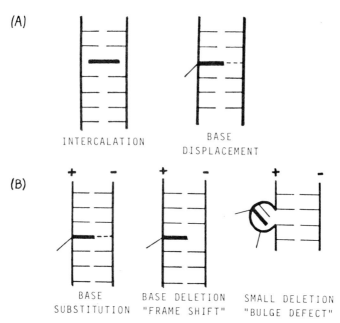

FIG. 3. (A) Schematic representation of a double-stranded nucleic acid with a planar drug, indicated by heavy line, inserted via intercalation or via base displacement. The vertical lines indicate
the nucleic acid backbone and the horizontal lines complementary base pairs between the two
strands. (B) Schematic representation of types of mutation that might occur as a consequence of
the base displacement model. (+) designates a template strand during replication to which the
drug (heavy line) is attached, and (−) designates the daughter strand. (For additional details see
Levine et al: Cancer Res 34: 319–327, 1974; reproduced by permission.)

Figure 3(B) illustrates schematically a mechanism by which base displacement could produce frame shift and deletion type mutations. Ames has
indeed found that AAF derivatives are extremely potent frame shift
mutagens in *Salmonella Typhimurium* and AAF has been reported to
induce deletions in *Drosophila* by the Fahmys. The *in vivo* consequences of
AAF modification of DNA will of course also be a function of the
responses of different polymerases and nucleases and the efficiency and
fidelity of DNA repair mechanisms.

Finally, despite the simplicity of the mutation theory of carcinogenesis, I
must emphasize that at the present time it is not clear whether AAF (or any
other carcinogen) causes the conversion of a normal cell to a tumor cell by:
(1) inducing mutations and/or chromosomal abnormalities; (2) influencing
cell selection, for example by suppressing immunologic surveillance or other
host defense mechanisms; (3) activating or enhancing the activity of viruses
or virus-related genes; or (4) inducing aberrations in differentiation at the

epigenetic level. Evidence related to each of these possibilities has been recently summarized elsewhere (Weinstein, Yamaguchi and Gebert, 1975). Table 6 lists current evidence favoring either the somatic mutation or the aberrant differentiation theories of carcinogenesis.

It is apparent that none of the current evidence is decisive. Personally I am impressed with the broad disturbances in the control of gene expression manifest by tumors as well as the increasing number of examples demonstrating the capacity of tumor cells to "revert" to a more normal phenotype. Therefore, I favor the theory of aberrant differentiation. Hopefully, recent exciting advances in methodology in cell culture systems should facilitate elucidation of the actual mechanism of chemical carcinogenesis. The results could have profound implications in terms of both cancer prevention and treatment. If, for example, it is found that carcinogenesis is due to an aberration in differentiation and not a mutation then there will be a

TABLE 6. Evidence Favoring Somatic Mutation or Aberrant Differentiation as Mechanisms of Carcinogenesis

Somatic Mutation	Aberrant Differentiation
1. The tumor phenotype is stable.	1. Differentiation and/or commitment stable.
2. Carcinogens attack DNA.	2. a. Carcinogens attack RNA and protein. b. DNA binding and carcinogenicity correlate poorly.
3. Many carcinogens are mutagens.	3. a. Some mutagens are not carcinogens (base analogs, hydroxylamine, acridines). b. Carcinogens are teratogens. c. The efficiency of transformation in cell culture is higher than random mutation rates.
4. Defective DNA repair is associated with increased tumor incidence, e.g., in xeroderma pigmentosum.	4. Not all patients with xeroderma pigmentosum have defective DNA repair. Cause and effect relationship is not established. 5. Tumors display broad disturbance in gene expression (hormone synthesis, fetal genes, isozymes). 6. TS mutants, revertants, and teratomas suggest reversibility of the tumor phenotype.

(From Weinstein et al: *In Vitro* 11:130, 1975).

TABLE 7. Examples of Reversion or Redifferentiation of Tumor Cells

---

In the animal
1. Crowngall tumor (plant) grafted onto normal plant yields normal seeds.
2. Lücke renal carcinoma (frog) nuclei transplanted into enucleated egg yield embryos with well-differentiated tissues.
3. Anaplastic embryonal carcinoma (mouse) converts to highly differentiated teratoma.
4. Teratocarcinoma cells (mouse) transferred into recipient blastocysts participate in the formation of a normal mouse.
5. In endometrial carcinoma (human) progesterone induces formation of decidua and secretory glands in the tumor.
6. Neuroblastoma (human) may regress or convert to ganglioneuromas.
7. Hormone-induced regression of breast, prostate, and uterine cancer (human).

In cell culture
1. Reversion of virus or chemically transformed cells to "normal" cells.
2. Reversible change in transformed cell phenotype in temperature-sensitive mutants.
3. Differentiation of leukemia cells into macrophages and granulocytes.
4. DMSO induction of hemoglobin synthesis in erythroleukemia cells.
5. Induction of phenotypic reversion by cAMP, BUdR and glucocorticoids.

---

sound theoretical basis for approaches to cancer therapy which include the design of agents that "re-program" tumor cells so that they either: (1) revert to a more normal growth pattern, (2) assume a growth pattern which normal host-defense or tissue involution mechanisms will respond to, or (3) pass into a pattern of terminal differentiation. Just to indicate that these ideas are not too far out, I have listed in Table 7 current examples of such phenomena. These examples indicate that at least certain cancer cells retain most if not all of the information present in normal cells and that under appropriate circumstances the pattern of gene expression and state of differentiation of cancer cells can be reprogrammed.

ACKNOWLEDGMENTS: The author wishes to acknowledge the invaluable collaboration he has had in these studies with Drs. Dezider Grunberger, Charles Cantor, Louis Fink, Louis Katz, James Nelson, Steven Blobstein, Concetta Pietropaolo and Mrs. Augusta Levine.

This work was supported by U.S.P.H.S. Research Grant CA-02332, and Contract E-72-3234 and The Alma Toorock Memorial for Cancer Research.

RELATED REFERENCES

Grungerger D, Weinstein IB: *In* Yuhas JM, Tennant RW, Regan JB (Eds): Biology of Radiation Carcinogens. New York, Raven Press, 1976.

Heidelberger C: Chemical carcinogenesis. *In* Ann Rev Biochem p. 79, 1975.

Miller JA: Cancer Res 30: 559, 1970.

Pietropaolo C, Weinstein IB: Cancer Res 35: 1291, 1975.

Pott P: Chirurgical Observations Relative to the Cataract, the Polypus of the Nose, the Cancer of the Scrotum, the Different Kinds of Ruptures and Mortification of the Toes and Feet. London, Hawes, Clarke and Collins, 1975, p. 208.

Sarma DSR, Rajalakshmi S, Farber E: *In* Becker FF (Ed.): Cancer: A Comprehensive Treatise, Vol. 1. New York, Plenum, 1975.

Weinstein IB, Grunberger D: *In* Ts'o POP, DiPaolo JA (Eds.): Chemical Carcinogenesis. New York, Marcel Dekker, 1974, p. 217.

Weinstein IB, Grunberger D, Blobstein S: Conformational and functional changes in nucleic acids induced by chemical carcinogens. Excerpta Medica International Congress Series No. 350, Vol. 2, Chemical and Viral Oncogenesis. Proceedings of the XI International Cancer Congress, Florence, 1974, Amsterdam, Excerpta Medica, 1974.

Weinstein IB, Yamaguchi N, Gebert R: In Vitro 11: 130, 1975.

Weisburger JH, Williams GM: *In* Becker FF (Ed): Cancer Vol. 1. New York, Plenum, 1975, p. 185.

Recent and Potential Advances in Cancer Chemotheraphy

Joseph H. Burchenal, M.D.

DISCOVERIES LEADING TO CANCER THERAPY

In discussing the recent and potential advances in cancer therapy, it is important to consider what made these possible. I submit that most advances came about in large part when and because they were believed to be eventually achievable. I would like to trace some of the events which I believe led to the present advances. The chemotherapy of cancer and of infectious disease have been closely intertwined and the advances in the chemotherapy of cancer have been, for the most part, based on advances in the treatment of infectious disease [4]. The demonstration over 300 years ago that a tea made from the bark of the chinchona tree could be used to treat malaria was the first instance of a specific chemotherapy against infectious disease. This was followed over two centuries later by the systematic studies of Ehrlich [16,17], which led to drugs effective against trypanosomes, and finally against the spirochete of syphilis, as well as the dye, methylene blue, weakly effective against malaria. Stimulated by the work of Ehrlich, Mietsch and Domagk [13,14] screened a series of dyes against various infectious disease organisms, including the hemolytic streptococcus, and found a red dye, prontosil, which would protect the mice against this infection. This was rapidly translated to the clinical sphere, with cures of puerperal sepsis, streptococcal septicemia and streptococcal meningitis. This proved that the chemotherapy of infectious diseases of bacterial origin was indeed possible, and led to the resurrection of Fleming's [27] original discovery of the inhibitory effect of an extract of penicillium on the *Staphylococcus aureus*. The active moiety of prontosil was found to be paraaminobenzenesulfonamide or sulfanilamide [59]. This in turn was found to act as an atagonist of paraaminobenzoic acid and this led to the formulation of the theory of antimetabolites by Woods [67] and Fildes [25]. The tremendous success of penicillin in the treatment of war wounds put chemo-

From the Memorial Sloan-Kettering Cancer Center, New York, N.Y.

Acknowledgement of support: NCI Grant CA-08748, United Leukemia Fund, ACS CI-116-Q, Alexandra Montgomery Fund, Hearst Foundation, and CCRC Grant CA-05826-14

therapy on a firm footing, and investigators realized that one could develop agents with a selectivity against disease processes. Thus, the investigators in the Chemical Warfare Service, noting that the nitrogen mustard, methyl-bis-(β-chloroethyl)-amine, caused destruction of normal lymphoid and bone marrow tissues in animals exposed to toxicity, postulated that this might have even more effect on diseases where there was an overgrowth of the lymphoid system, such as lymphosarcoma and leukemia [31]. This, indeed, turned out to be the case, and led to the tremendous number of alkylating agents which have appeared on the horizon over the past 30 years—some great improvements over the original compounds.

The theory of antimetabolites led to the folic acid antoagonists, aminopterin and methotrexate, in the treatment of leukemia [24] and now as part of combination therapy for many different carcinomas and sarcomas, and also to the classic studies of Hitchings and Elion [18–20,33], which in turn gave us such diverse compounds as 6-mercaptopurine, thioguanine, allopurinol, azathioprine and pyrimethamine. These, in turn, led to the discoveries of the arabinosyl pyrimidines [22,62] and the azapyrimidines [40a,48], both useful in the treatment of acute myeloblastic leukemia.

From the antibiotic filtrates have derived such compounds as actinomycin D [62], so effective in choriocarcinoma of the uterus [40] and useful in the combination therapy of testicular tumors [42], Daunomycin [11], a very useful agent in the treatment of AML [2,57] and, to a lesser degree, in ALL, and its congener, Adriamycin [12], which is not only active in the leukemias and the lymphomas, but also is perhaps the best antibiotic available for the treatment, particularly in combination, of the sarcomas and carcinomas. Bleomycin is another active agent differing from the other antitumor antibiotics in having no bone marrow suppressive toxicity [60,61].

Among the compounds derived from natural sources, there are many that are effective in experimental, and a few in clinical, studies. Among the most important are those derived from the Vinca alkaloids: vinblastine, which is of great value in Hodgkin's disease, and vincristine, which is extremely valuable in the remission induction in acute leukemias [21], and is also used in many different combinations in solid tumors. A new derivative of these, desacetyl vinblastine amide sulfate, with different toxicities from vincristine and vinblastine, is now under study.

In addition to these main lines of research, new compounds have appeared, sometimes at random, sometimes as intermediates in the synthesis of some desired compound, which, during screening, have turned out to possess experimental and clinical antitumor activity. Procarbazine [5] and dimethyl-triazeno-imidazole-carboxamide (DTIC) [54] are examples of this type. As more and more success is achieved in chemotherapy, as the screening methods are improved, and as the molecular areas of activity are better defined, more and more new agents are becoming available for clinical testing each year.

ACCESSION OF NEW DRUGS

The ideal and more intellectually satisfying situation would be to determine differences between the cancer cell and the most sensitive vital normal cells in enzyme content, or nutritional requirements, and on the basis of these differences to design compounds selectively effective against the cancer cell. We know of few such differences, however, and in the accession of new agents, it is obvious that screening technics are of the utmost importance. Practical predictive models for detecting activity of compounds against human cancer must be considered not only on the ability of the technic to predict, but also on the cost and the ease with which they can be used. The least expensive form of predictive mechanism would presumably be mouse or human tumor or leukemic cells in tissue culture or even bacteria in culture [26]. Unfortunately, such systems detect general cytotoxicity and do not differentiate between toxicity to the tumor cells versus the normal cells. While they will usually detect very toxic active agents, they give occasional false positives because the rapid excretion and rapid metabolism of some compounds *in vivo* is not taken into consideration in the *in vitro* tests. They can also give false negative results occasionally in compounds such as cyclophosphamide, which must be metabolized to active derivatives in the liver, and are relatively inactive *in vitro,* in contrast to their great activity *in vivo*. Thus, although *in vitro* tests are valuable indicators because of the small amount of compound required, and because of their extreme sensitivity, the *in vitro* method should be used only as a very preliminary indication of the activity of compounds, and should always be supplemented with *in vivo* studies.

In vivo models on the other hand have built-in toxicity controls with many sensitive, vital normal tissues, such as the bone marrow, gut epithelium, kidney and liver [26]. Thus, they are able to demonstrate a chemotherapeutic activity as contrasted to a purely toxic effect, and can give the therapeutic index of a drug. *In vivo* predictive models are largely limited to the mouse, rat, and guinea pig. Because of the expense involved, and the ease of handling, as well as the fact that there are many more inbred lines, the mouse is generally the experimental animal of choice. One must then decide whether to use spontaneous, induced, or transplanted tumors or leukemias.

Inbred mouse strains such as the AKR and C58 have a very high incidence of spontaneous lymphoid leukemia in older mice. Certain others, such as the C3H, have a high incidence of mammary tumors; but these spontaneous leukemias and tumors require a large colony of old mice in order to supply sufficient spontaneous tumors for a screening program and are not generally as predictable in time of survival following diagnosis as are the transplanted leukemias and tumors.

A high incidence of tumors may be induced in some strains of mice and rats by carcinogens, and these can also be used for screening. Although they have special areas of usefulness, such as detecting anticarcinogenic effects and immunologic or chemotherapeutic effects on the very early tumor, they have many of the drawbacks of the spontaneous tumors and leukemias.

Transplanted L1210 leukemia in the mouse has been extremely satisfactory in predicting agents with activity in acute myeloid and acute lymphoid leukemia in man, as well as activity against certain other lymphomas and few other tumors [26]. The compounds active against L1210, however, are less often of great value in the treatment of such carcinomas as those of the lung, colon, pancreas and breast, and for this reason, transplanted tumors, such as the Lewis lung carcinoma, the mouse mammary carcinoma 26, the colon carcinoma 44, the B16 melanoma and the Ridgway Osteogenic Sarcoma, are also used as screening agents for their effects against solid tumors. These tumors are particularly useful in that one can correlate the effects of a drug with the size of the tumor and can also demonstrate the enhanced effects of these compounds when used immediately after local surgery has removed the bulk of the tumor.

A good example of the various data that can be derived from studies on one of these tumors is shown in Figure 1 [52], in which it can be seen with this advanced mammary tumor that (1) surgery alone is unable to cure the animal because presumably the tumor has already metastasized beyond the field of surgery; (2) chemotherapy alone is unable to cure the animal because the bulk of the tumor is too large and, although therapy may destroy several logs of cells, it cannot destroy enough to bring about a cure; (3) when, however, the great bulk of the tumor is removed by surgery and full doses of the combination are given, it is possible to cure a large percentage of the animals; (4) this same technic, of adjuvant therapy employing only two-thirds of the dose of the drug combination, however, is much less effective. Thus, this demonstrates the weaknesses of both surgery and chemotherapy when used alone, the advantages of adjuvant chemotherapy immediately following surgery, and the dangers inherent on decreasing from the maximum tolerated dose of chemotherapy.

Mechanism of action studies attempting to block the inhibitory effect of a given agent against tumors or leukemic cells, can be done in tissue culture or in the intact animal. These give, in some instances, a clear indication of

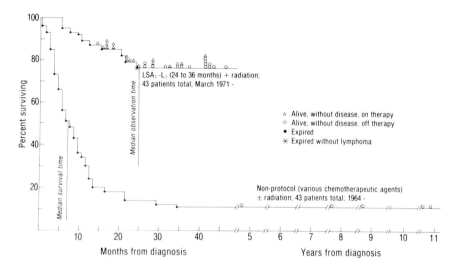

FIG. 1. Non-Hodgkin's Lymphoma in Children: 1964–January 31, 1975 (86 patients total).

how compounds are working. In some cases, notably high-dose methotrexate followed by citrovorum factor, such studies have allowed a much larger dose of the therapeutic agent to be given and still have the toxicity protected against by citrovorum factor. This had led to the outstanding results which we will discuss later in certain of the solid tumors in man.

Cell kinetic studies are important in determining the percentage of cells in the proliferative phase in a given tumor as contrasted to those in the resting stage. This growth fraction has important implications as to therapy, since cell cycle-specific agents are more effective against tumors with a high percentage of cells in the proliferating phase (high growth fraction) as contrasted to tumors with a low growth fraction, which are generally better treated by cycle nonspecific agents.

RECENT ADVANCES IN THERAPY

Early clinical trial rapidly demonstrated the activity of a large number of single agents against various types of tumors and leukemias. With the exception of choriocarcinoma of the uterus [41] and Burkitt's tumor [7,44,68], cures were not achieved with single agent therapy, however; this was not until the efficacy of combination therapy was demonstrated first by Bernard [3] with methotrexate and cortisone, and later, and perhaps more importantly, with intensive intermittent combination therapy by Freireich,

Karon and Frei [28] in the VAMP Protocol in acute leukemia. It was immediately following this and the MOPP Protocol by De Vita et al. [10,45] in Stage III and IV Hodgkin's Disease, that combination therapy really came into its own and began to achieve long-term survivors and presumably occasional cures.

Hematologic Neoplasms

Spectacular advances have been made in the last 10 years in the treatment of the hematologic neoplasms. This stems primarily from the use of intensive intermittent combination chemotherapy plus prophylaxis of the CNS involvement in leukemias by radiation, intrathecal methotrexate, or 1-B-D-arabinofuranosylcytosine (ara-C) [29,32,46]. In acute lymphoblastic leukemia in children, complete remissions can be achieved in approximately 95% of the patients with vincristine and prednisone, induced frequently with the addition of Adriamycin or Daunomycin or asparaginase. Prophylaxis of the meningeal involvement is then achieved with either cranio-spinal radiation or cranial radiation plus intrathecal methotrexate, or intrathecal methotrexate, with or without ara-C, but without radiation. A short course of consolidation therapy is often given, consisting of ara-C and thioguanine or 5-day courses of methotrexate. Maintenance therapy is then continued for 3 years with daily mercaptopurine, weekly methotrexate, interspersed with reinduction regimens of vincristine and prednisone, or some of the non-cycle-specific agents such as actinomycin-D, bis (β-chloroethyl) nitrosourea (BCNU), Cytoxan, or Adriamycin. There are many such regimens being used at the present time and most of these project that at least 50% of the patients will remain in their initial remission, free of disease at 5 years. Presumably, most of these will not relapse.

In acute nonlymphoblastic leukemia which occurs mainly in adults, the results have not been nearly so satisfying. Most of the treatment regimens are based on ara-c, usually combined with either thioguanine, Daunomycin, or Adriamycin. Ara-C, because of its short half-life, must be given every 12 hours, every 8 hours, or by continuous administration. With most of the regimens employing these drugs, anywhere from 50 to 70% complete remissions may be achieved. Following this, maintenance therapy is continued for 1 to 2, sometimes 3 years, with either repeated courses of the inducing agent or a combination of 4 days of a cycle-specific agent followed immediately by injection of a non-cycle-specific agent, every 2 to 3 weeks. Recently, two new derivatives of ara-C, 2,2´-anhydro-1-B-D-arabinofuranosylcytosine (AAC) (cyclocytidine) [34], or 2,2´-anhydro-1-B-D-arabinofuranosyl-5-flurocytosine (AAFC) [28], have been shown to be

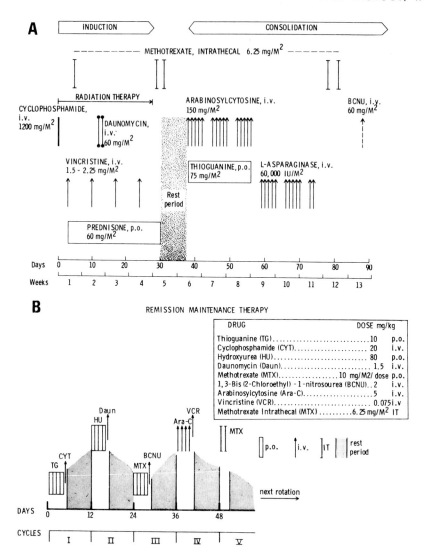

FIG. 2. (A) Intensive Chemotherapy for Lymphosarcoma and Reticulum Cell Sarcoma in Children: LSA-2 (L2) Protocol. (B) Intensive Chemotherapy for Acute Lymphoblastic Leukemia and Leukosarcoma in Children and Adults (L-2 Protocol).

more effective in mouse leukemia and to have longer half-lives in man than ara-C. Both of these compounds are under preliminary study at the present time and will produce approximately 50% remissions in patients with acute nonlymphoblastic leukemia. AAFC appears to produce remissions more rapidly, usually after the first course, and to produce less nausea and vomiting than ara-C, but further study will be required to determine whether it has any significant advantages over ara-C [2].

In Stage III and IV Hodgkin's disease, the MOPP program as started by De Vita et al. [10,45], using nitrogen mustard, vincristine, procarbazine, and prednisone, in short courses lasting 2 weeks out of every 4 for a total of 6 courses, has produced approximately 50% patients with no evidence of disease after 5 years. Attempts are now being made to improve these results by continuing maintenance therapy with wider spaced courses of MOPP or with other agents. In addition, an intensive protocol using four active but different drugs has been used by Bonadonna [6] with excellent results in patients whose disease has become resistant to the MOPP regimen. Kaplan and Rosenberg are also studying the effects of total nodal radiation followed by MOPP for Stage III and IV Hodgkin's disease.

The treatment of non-Hodgkin's lymphoma in children has been improved enormously by the regimen developed by Wollner et al. [64] in which a large dose of Cytoxan is followed immediately by radiation to the bulk of the tumor and the further induction of remission by a protocol (L2) designed for the treatment of acute lymphoblastic leukemia consisting of vincristine and prednisone and Adriamycin for induction, intrathecal methotrexate, consolidation with ara-C, and thioguanine, asparaginase, and BCNU, and then maintenance therapy for two years with cycle-specific and non-cycle-specific agents (Figs. 2A and 2B). The results of this regimen compared to historical controls are seen in Figure 3.

Solid Tumors in Children and Young Adults

Early treatment of these tumors with surgery or obliterative radiotherapy will obviously cure many patients, but, equally obviously, many have recur-

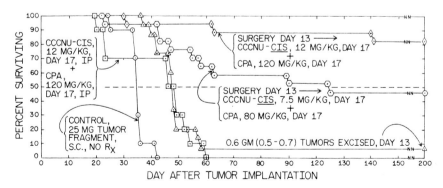

FIG. 3. C3H Mammary Tumor Line 44 in B_6C3F_1Mice

rences. If the chemotherapist waits until they have become clinically apparent, he will cure none. For this reason in most patients with solid tumors, multidisciplinary therapy will be considered.

Let us examine the experimental data from a number of investigations that provide the basis of adjuvant therapy with solid tumors such as Ca 755. Martin et al. [43] have shown that small tumors at 1 to 7 days after inoculation can be cured by chemotherapy, whereas the large 15-day tumor cannot. Schwartz et al. [53] have reported total regression and cure of Ridgway osteogenic sarcoma (ROS) with actinomycin D when tumors were about one gram at time of treatment Schabel [52] has reported marked reduction in actinomycin D and sarcolysin (L-PAM) activity against ROS if treatment is delayed until tumors are 2 to 4 grams in size. Another important fact to bear in mind is that, in mice, the most effective dose of most drugs or combinations is the maximum tolerated dose and decreases in dosage of even 20 to 33% may seriously compromise the therapeutic effect. In Ridgway osteogenic sarcoma, for example, a single dose of 10 mg/kg of L-PAM on day 12 is curative, but $\frac{2}{3}$ of that dose, 6.7 mg/kg, has almost no effect. Cyclophosphamide and even 5-fluorouracil lose much of their activity at $\frac{2}{3}$ of the maximum tolerated dose. As demonstrated in many tumors, certain combinations are also more effective than the maximum tolerated dose of either compound alone. Martin et al. [43] showed many years ago that if a tumor such as adenocarcinoma 755 is injected subcutaneously into mice and is allowed to grow for 15 days, surgery alone or chemotherapy alone will not cure the animal. If, however, surgery and chemotherapy are employed together, with the large primary tumor being excised surgically and the tiny pulmonary metastases being destroyed by chemotherapy, over half the animals survive. Similar results have been reported by Schabel, Griswold, Corbett, and Dykes [52,53] of Southern Research Institute with a spectrum of transplantable and metastasizing solid tumors—C3H mammary carcinoma (Fig. 3), Lewis lung carcinoma, colon carcinoma, and B16 melanoma—with the best results being achieved by full-dose intensive chemotherapy, frequently with combinations of drugs following surgical procedures. Smaller doses are likely to be less effective (Fig. 3).

If we now proceed from tumors in mice to tumors in children, we find the same principles are applicable. Wilms' tumor gave the first indication of the value of multidisciplinary therapy. Klapproth [39] reviewed the literature on Wilms' tumor from 1940 to 1958 and reported the cure rate with surgery with or without radiotherapy to be 17 to 23%, whereas Farber and his group [23], using surgery, radiotherapy and chemotherapy with actinomycin-D given almost simultaneously, followed by repeated courses of actinomycin-D every three months, reported an 80% cure rate in this previously highly incurable disease. Even in Wilms' tumor with pulmonary metastases, the combination of radiotherapy and actinomycin-D has produced approximately 50% long-term, disease-free survival [23].

In Ewing's tumor, as has been previously mentioned, we have a neoplasm which is highly sensitive to radiation therapy and also relatively responsive to chemotherapy. If in the early case, however, the primary tumor is treated with only radiation therapy in full therapeutic doses, 5000 to 7000 rads tumor dose, the primary will be completely eradicated, but 80 to 90% of the patients will go on to die of metastases elsewhere, even though they appeared to be completely free of disease other than the primary tumor at the time radiation therapy was given. Similarly, if one treats with chemotherapy only after the appearance of metastases, considerable regression can be obtained. Such regressions are temporary, however, and total cures are rarely obtained. If, however, the therapeutic dose of radiation therapy is given to the primary tumor and this is followed immediately by adjuvant chemotherapy with the combination of cyclophosphamide and vincristine, with or without actinomycin-D and adriamycin, good results have been achieved, ranging between 55 and 70% long-term disease-free survivals, many of which are presumed to be cures [35,49].

In embryonal rhadomyosarcoma, a disease which is less sensitive to radiotherapy and somewhat less sensitive to chemotherapy also, multidisciplinary therapy—with surgery to remove the bulk of the tumor, radiation to destroy any tumor that cannot be removed surgically and intensive combination chemotherapy with the same four agents mentioned above for the micrometastases—has produced exciting results, with marked increase in long-term disease-free survival [15,30,48]. Ghavimi et al. recently have reported 21 of 25 patients NED, and in the intervening 12 months none of these has relapsed (Table 1). The results of these and other investigators

TABLE 1. Embryonal Rhabdomyosarcoma

Author	Type	Surgery, Radiation and Chemotherapy	Duration of Therapy	Complete Remissions	NED	Duration of Remissions
Pratt	All	VCR, CTX, Act.-D	6–12 mos.		15/34	30+–75+ mos. (19)
Wilbur	Head & Neck	VCR, CTX, Act.-D	24 mos.		13/19	48+–132+ mos. (5, 30)
Ghavimi	All	VCR, CTX, Act.-D Adria.	24 mos.		21/25	9 for 36+–48+ mos. 12 for 24+–36+ mos. (7–8)

noted in Table 1, particularly those long-term NED patients of Wilbur, suggest that these are permanent cures.

Now let us progress to an even more difficult tumor to treat—osteogenic sarcoma. In the overt metastatic stage this tumor is relatively resistant to radiotherapy and is refractory to most ordinary forms of chemotherapy [38]. Here, too, surgery alone has a dismal track record [37]. The survival rate from radical surgery alone has varied little over the past twenty years, with approximately 50% of the patients developing pulmonary metastases between 5 and 9 months and 80% by 18 months after surgery and no better than 20% over-all five-year cures. But here, again, with radical surgery followed by adjuvant chemotherapy using various combinations of vincristine, high-dose methotrexate with CF rescue, adriamycin and cyclophosphamide [55], there has been a tremendous improvement in results (Table 2), with Jaffe and Frei et al. [36,37] reporting 75% (9 out of 12) patients free of disease for from 13 to 30 months after surgery, using as adjuvant therapy only vincristine and high-dose methotrexate with CF rescue. Cortes et al.

TABLE 2. Results of Surgery Plus Adjuvant Chemotherapy in Primary
Osteogenic Sarcoma

Investigator	Chemotherapy	Duration Rx (mos.)	Eval.	NED	Duration (mos.)
Pratt et al.	Adria., HDMTX, CTX	10	5	4	19+ to 26+
Sutow et al.	CTX, VCR Sarcolysin Adria.	16	18	10	32+ to 47+
Jaffe, Frei et al.	HDMTX	24	12	9	12+ to 30+
Cortes, Holland et al.	Adria.	6	13	10	13+ to 44+
Rosen et al.	VCR, HDMTX, CTX, Adria.				
	1. with amputation	12	11	9	3+ to 14+
	2. with bone replacement	12	14	13	4+ to 17+
	3. with amputation* and thoracotomy	12	11	10	6+ to 31+

* 2/10 had bone replacement prior to thoracotomy, 1 of whom had operable pulm. mets. (May 15, 1975).

[8,9], in those patients in whom maximum tolerated doses of adriamycin alone followed radical surgery, have 10 of the 13 cases originally reported surviving, with no evidence of disease 13 to 44 months after surgery.

The most important series is the adjuvant therapy of osteogenic sarcoma, however, is that of Sutow et al. [56] (COMPADRI I) (Table 2). They reported that 10 of 18 patients were NED more than 19 months after surgery. These 10 patients remain NED now 32 to 47 months after surgery and 16 to 31 months after discontinuance of adjuvant therapy. These 10 cases would now appear to be true cures of the disease. If such results can be achieved with a tumor as refractory to surgery, radiotherapy or chemotherapy as osteogenic sarcoma, it would seem reasonable to expect at least as good results with the solid tumors of adults.

These, then, are the Basic Principles of Adjuvant Therapy [8]:

1. Surgery and radiation therapy are limited not by the size of the tumor, but by its extension, whereas chemotherapy and immunotherapy are limited not by the extension of the tumor but by its total mass.

2. Chemotherapy is most effective when given at the maximum tolerated dose; combination therapy is usually better than treatment with single drugs, and mild low-dose chemotherapy may be ineffective.

3. Adjuvant therapy should be given as soon as possible after surgery in order to destroy the vulnerable micrometastases before they become macroscopic and relatively insensitive.

A particularly exciting multidisciplinary program for the treatment of osteogenic sarcoma is being studied by Rosen and Marcove [50]. This consists of two preoperative courses of intensive combination therapy with vincristine, high-dose methotrexate with CF rescue and adriamycin, followed by surgical removal of the tumor and complete replacement [55] of the affected bone by a metal prosthesis while preserving the nerves, vessels and most of the muscles, followed by postoperative adjuvant chemotherapy with the same drugs plus cyclophosphamide for 12 months. So far, twenty patients have been entered on this protocol, 14 have been operated on, and only one has, as yet, shown any evidence of recurrent disease after surgery. The longest, however, is still only 17 months postsurgery (Table 2).

The data from the five children's tumors that have been successfully treated by adjuvant therapy suggest that aggressive chemotherapy, which with a large tumor mass is only temporarily palliative, may be curative when there is minimal residual tumor. Thus, in adults, carcinoma of the breast with positive axillary nodes may be the ideal set-up for multidisciplinary therapy because we have many drugs and combinations which are active in the advanced disease. Carcinoma of the colon with local nodal involvement may be next, with a greater need of chemotherapeutic help but a lesser array of drugs to rely on. The recent exciting results in metastatic gastric disease reported by Moertel et al. with MeCCNU and 5-FU suggest one regimen that might be employed as adjuvant therapy. Stage II melanoma has an equally great need, even fewer strongly active drugs, and may be benefited occasionally by adjuvant immunotherapy. In carcinoma of the lung where the need of adjuvant therapy is almost absolute, we have the weakest effects to be expected at present from either chemotherapy or immunotherapy, and we must hit hardest with intensive intermittent combination chemotherapy. Perhaps here therapy of the type used in osteogenic sarcoma with vincristine, high dose methotrexate with Citrovorum Factor rescue (CF) and adriamycin might be of value. Certainly in this disease, as in osteogenic sarcoma, the most agressive, intensive adjuvant therapy is justified.

Bone Marrow Transplantation

In leukemias resistant to chemotherapy in which there is an HLA matched sibling, bone marrow transplants, after cytoreductive therapy, large doses of cytoxan, and total body irradiation, have been successful in producing about 30% long-term remissions in the hands of Thomas and his group [44a]. This is a laborious process, requiring a great deal of hospitalization and nursing care, and is fraught with great danger of graft versus host reaction and infection with opportunistic organisms. With improvements in the technic of marrow transplantation, better control of the graft versus host reactions and better anti-viral chemotherapy, however, this may assume considerable importance in the treatment of leukemias.

A similar situation may exist with the chemotherapy of solid tumors, where the aspiration and freezing of the patient's own bone marrow, followed by very high and otherwise lethal dose of chemotherapy and radiation, may suffice to destroy the last vestiges of the solid tumor, and the patient may be rescued by reinfusion of his previously stored marrow. Both of these technics are being explored by several different groups and may turn out to be of great value in the future in cases not responding to standard surgery or radiation, multidisciplinary adjuvant therapy, or to chemotherapy or immunotherapy of the advanced disease.

In summary, then, the chemotherapy of cancer has made great progress in the past 30 years. By and large the progress has consisted of many small steps rather than any major single breakthrough. The combined use with the other presently available modalities of intensive intermittent combination chemotherapy as adjuvant therapy may well represent, however, the greatest advance in the long history of the treatment of cancer.

REFERENCES

1. Armstrong JB, Dyke RA, Fouts PJ, Gahimer JE: Cancer Chemother Rep 18: 49, 1962.
2. Bernard J: Cancer Res 27: 2565, 1967.
3. Bernard J, Marie J, Salet J, Cruciani C: Bull Mem Soc Med Hopitaux 16: 621, 1951.
4. Bertino JR, Levitt M, McCullough JL, Chabner B: Ann NY Acad Sci 186: 486, 1971.
5. Bollag W, Grunberg E: Experientia 19: 130, 1963.
6. Bonadonna G, DeLena M, Uslenghi E, Zacali R: Proc Soc Clin Oncol 15: 90, 1974 (abstr).
7. Burkitt DP: Chemotherapy of jaw tumors. In Burchenal JH, Burkitt DP (Eds): Treatment of Burkitt's Tumor. Berlin, Springer, 1967, p 94.
8. Cortes E, Holland J, Wang J, et al: N Engl J Med 291: 998, 1974.
9. Cortes E: Personal communication.
10. DeVita VT Jr, Serpick A: Proc Am Assoc Cancer Res 8: 13 1967 (abstr).
11. DiMarco A, Gaetani M, Dorigotti L, et al: Cancer Chemother Rep 38: 31, 1964.
12. DiMarco A, Gaetani M, Scarpinato B: Cancer Chemother Rep 53: 33, 1969.
13. Donagk G: Dtsch Med wochenschr 61: 250, 1935.
14. Domagk G: Dtsch Med Wochenschr 61: 829, 1935.
15. Donaldson SS, Castro JR, Wilbur JR, Jesse RH Jr: Cancer 31: 2626, 1973, and personal communication.
16. Ehrlich P: Die Behandlung der Syphilis mit dem Ehrlichschen Praparat 606. Verh. 82. Vers Ges Dtsch Naturf Arzt, 1910.
17. Ehrlich P, Shiga K: Klin Wochenschr 41: 329, 1904.
18. Elion GB, Burgi E, Hitchings GH: J Am Chem Soc 74: 411, 1962.
19. Elion GB, Hitchings GH: J Am Chem Soc 77: 1676, 1955.
20. Elion GB, Hitchings GH, Van der Werff H: Purines. J Biol Chem 192: 505, 1951.
21. Evans AE: Cancer Chemother Rep 52: 469, 1968.
22. Evans JS, Musser EA, Bostwick L, Nengel GD: Cancer Res 24: 1285, 1964.
23. Farber S: JAMA 198: 826, 1966.
24. Farber S, Diamond LK, Mercer RD, et al: N Engl J Med 238: 787, 1948.
25. Fildes P: Lancet 1: 955, 1940.
26. Fischer GA: Ann NY Acad Sci 76: 673, 1958.
27. Fleming A: Br J Exp Pathol 10: 226, 1929.
28. Fox JJ, Falco EA, Wempen I, et al: Cancer Res 32: 2269, 1972.
29. Freireich EJ, Karon M, Frei E III: Proc Am Assoc Cancer Res 5: 20, 1964 (abstr).
30. George P, Hernandez K, Hustu O, et al: J Pediat 72: 399, 1968.
31. Ghavimi F, Exelby P, D'Angio G, et al: Cancer 35: 677, 1975.
32. Gilman A, Goodman L, Lindskog GE, Dougherty S: Science 103: 409, 1946.
33. Haghbin M, Tan CC, Clarkson BD, et al: Cancer 33; 1491, 1974.
34. Hitchings GH, Rhoads CP: Ann NY Acad Sci 60: 183, 1954.
35. Hoshi A, Kanzawa F, Kuretani K, et al: Gann 62: 145, 1971.
36. Hustu HO, Pinkel D, Pratt CB: Cancer 30: 1522, 1972.
37. Jaffe N, Frei E: Personal communication.
38. Jaffe N, Frei E, Traggis D, Bishop Y: N Engl J Med 291: 994, 1974.
39. Jaffe N, Paed D: Cancer 30: 1627, 1972.
40. Klapproth HJ: J Urol 81: 633, 1959.
41. Karon J, Sieger L, Leimbrock S, et al: Proc Am Assoc Cancer Res 14: 94 #373, 1973.
42. Li MC: Med Clin North Am 45: 661, 1961.
43. Li MC, Hertz R, Spencer DB: Proc Soc Exp Biol Med 93: 361, 1956.
44. Li MC, Whitmore WF Jr, Gilbey R, Grabstald H: JAMA 174: 1291, 1960.
45. Martin DS, Fugmann RA: Cancer Res 17: 1098, 1957.

46. Oettgen HF, Burkitt D, Burchenal JH: Cancer 16:616, 1963.
47. Perry S, Thomas LB, Johnson RE, et al: Ann Intern Med 67: 424, 1967.
48. Pinkel D: JAMA 216: 648, 1971.
49. Piskala A, Sorm F: Coll Czech Chem Commun 29: 2060–2076, 1964.
50. Pratt CB, Hustu HO, Fleming ID, Pinkel D: Cancer Res 32: 606, 1972.
51. Rosen G, Wollner N, Wu S, et al: 26th Annual James Ewing Society Meeting, Abstract #23, 1973.
52. Neiman P, Thomas ED, Buekner CD, et al: Ann Rev Med 25: 179–198, 1974.
53. Rosen G, Murphy M, Marcove R: Proc James Ewing Society, March 1975.
54. Schabel FM Jr: *In* Cancer Chemotherapy—Fundamental Concepts and Recent Advances. Chicago, Year Book, 1975, pp 323–355.
55. Schwartz HS, Sodergren JE, Sternberg SS, Philips FS: Cancer Res 26: 1873, 1966.
56. Shealy YF, Montgomery JA, Laster WR Jr: Biochem Pharmacol 11: 674, 1962.
57. Sutow WW: Personal communication.
58. Sutow WW, Sullivan MP, Fernback DJ: Proc Am Assoc Cancer Res 15: 20, 1974.
59. Tan C, Tosaka H, You KP, et al: Cancer 20: 333, 1967.
60. Trefouel J, Trefouel J, Nitti F, Bovet D: C R Soc Biol (Paris) 120: 756, 1935.
61. Umezawa H: *In* Holland J, Frei E (Eds): Cancer Medicine. Philadelphia, Lea and Fegiber, 1973, p 817.
62. Umezawa H, Maeda K, Takeuchi T, Okami Y: J Antibiot (Tokyo) 19: 200, 1966.
63. Waksman S, Woodruff HB: Proc Soc Exp Biol Med 45: 609, 1940.
64. Walwick ER, Dekker CA; Roberts WK: Proc Chem Soc 1959, p 84.
65. Wollner N, Burchenal JH, Lieberman P, et al: J Med Ped Oncol 1975 (in press).
66. Wollner N, Burchenal JH, Lieberman P, et al: Cancer 1975 (in press).
67. Wollner N, D'Angio G, Burchenal JH, et al: Proc Am Assoc Cancer Res 14: 97, 1973 (abstr).
68. Woods DD: Br J Exp Pathol 21: 74, 1940.
69. Ziegler JL: Cancer 30: 1534, 1972.